The Medical School Coach

Waking Your Inner Doctor

Gary Rose, M.D., F.A.C.S

Past Chairman of the Admissions Committee, University of Miami School of Medicine Regional Campus, Boca Raton, Florida

Member of the Admissions Committee, Charles E. Schmidt College of Medicine, Florida Atlantic University, Boca Raton, Florida

Co-Director of the Post-Baccalaureate Program, Charles E. Schmidt College of Medicine, Florida Atlantic University, Boca Raton, Florida

ISBN: 1502755912
ISBN 13: 9781502755919
Library of Congress Control Number: 2014918106
CreateSpace Independent Publishing Platform
North Charleston, South Carolina

What Others Are Saying

Dr. Rose's motivation, guidance, and mentorship were essential in my acceptance to medical school and progression into orthopedic surgery.
—*M. K. Smith, MD, orthopedic surgery resident*

"The advice in this book played an essential role in my acceptance to medical school. It is an absolute must-read for anyone serious about pursuing a career in medicine. If you're looking for an honest insider's perspective on the medical-school application process from a true authority, read *The Medical School Coach*."
—*E. Polcz, medical student*

"Any student on the premed track absolutely needs to read this book. Without the instructions and knowledge provided by Dr. Rose, I wouldn't have been accepted to medical school...I didn't know the first thing about applying to programs, and Dr. Rose took me from a hopeful undergrad to a competent medical student."
—*J. Miller, medical student*

"Dr. Rose has been extremely influential in my understanding and pursuit of the medical profession. His personal approach dispels many of the myths, misconceptions, and even superstitions so many of us premeds have. I have no doubt that this book will help me achieve my goal of getting into medical school."
—*D. Henry, premedical student*

To Ryan and Rachel, my children, who over the years have "listened" to all that I have written here. I am so proud of who they are becoming.

Acknowledgments

I wish to thank all of my teachers and all of my students. Each has played a role in helping me write, direct, and star in my "movie." They have inspired me throughout my lifetime and have led me to the path that I have followed. I also want to thank Donell Henry for his suggestions and Valerie Erica Polcz for her review, her re-reviews, and her assistance in shaping this book.

Contents

Foreword

As an internationally known Beverly Hills plastic surgeon and Emmy Award-winning talk show host, I have the opportunity to meet and talk with all kinds of people. New methods and techniques emerge daily. Many of them are here today and gone tomorrow. But every once in a while, I meet someone with a message that is a game-changer—someone who has a message that can change the way people think and do things. Gary Rose, MD, is one of those people—a changer with a powerful message.

I first met Gary many years ago. We have both given many presentations at national and international meetings and found ourselves as panelists at the same scientific session at one of the large international meetings. I knew Gary by reputation, and when I heard him speak with such passion and conviction, he got my attention. I couldn't help but listen to his message. Ever since that day, we have been good friends and have stayed in contact.

Later, Gary and I appeared together on a leading national television talk show. He stole the show that day, and our host, the audience, and I were all able to clearly see that Gary truly was an expert at delivering the message—his message.

As one of the "docs" on the Emmy Award-winning informational talk show *The Doctors*, I interact with many people who claim to be experts on all kinds of topics. Dr. Gary Rose is the "real deal," and he has proven it to me in the most direct way possible. When I asked Gary to help my son Matthew, he did just that. Gary used his years of experience as an admissions-committee member and chairman to advise Matt on getting into medical school. He helped Matt work with his strengths, develop his skills, and wisely plan out his medical-school admission strategies. I am so proud of Matt, who was accepted to multiple medical schools and is now in his third year at Keck School of Medicine at the University of Southern California (USC). I know that Gary's input and advice contributed significantly to my family's medical-school admission success.

Dr. Rose is very organized and clear in his approach to medical school acceptance. In fact, he is the "Medical School Coach." His humanistic, down-to-earth approach is the key to the success of his method. His conversations, and now the chapters in this book, empowered my son and the other premed students whom he has advised with the tools and information that they needed to develop into the best medical-school applicants possible. In addition, the information and advice contained within this book are extremely helpful for life.

I feel that *The Medical School Coach* should be a must-read for every young man and woman who desires to apply to medical school and become a doctor.

Andrew P. Ordon, MD, FACS
Certified American Board of Plastic Surgery
Certified American Board of Head and Neck Surgery
Host of the Emmy Award-winning TV show *The Doctors*
Assistant Adjunct Professor of Surgery
Dartmouth Medical School

Preface

This is truly a unique book that is directed to the millions of high-school and college-age students (and their parents) who desire to go to medical school. It will greatly help them realize their dream of being accepted into their schools of choice.

This is clearly not a manual or a how-to book. There are already a few out there, and they just tell you how to fill out the forms, what courses to take, and a summary of the statistics of medical schools in the United States. There honestly can't be a one-size-fits-all manual to tell you how to get into medical school.

This gem of a book is different—and much more exciting. It is a book that emphasizes how to acquire the attributes, characteristics, and consciousness that will make the medical-school applicant the absolute best candidate possible for acceptance into medical school in the United States.

Throughout the book, I illustrate major points with meaningful, interesting anecdotes that will emphasize and further teach you how to develop the qualities and traits that are most desirable and necessary to be accepted into medical school.

In fact, this is a book that will guide students to become the very best human beings they possibly can be. Most importantly, it is a book on self-improvement and will help guide you to develop and master the life skills that will improve your life and the lives of all of the people that you come in contact with.

As past chairman of the admissions committee of the University of Miami School of Medicine Regional Campus at Florida Atlantic University in Boca Raton, and then continuing as an active member of the admissions committee of the Charles E. Schmidt College of Medicine in Boca Raton, I have had many years of experience understanding and defining what it takes to get into medical school.

After interviewing hundreds of medical-school candidates and working with medical students for over a decade, I have learned what makes them tick.

This book is written in a style that relates to today's "sound-bite" society. It speaks to the computer generation in particular—short, cogent, and without fluff.

You can pick up this book and read any chapter, in or out of sequence, and still get the entire message.

I know that you will have as much enjoyment reading this book as I have had writing it.

Introduction

I write this book for every one of you who, for even a moment, had the thought, the idea, or ever even considered being a doctor. Perhaps becoming a doctor was just a passing fancy. In the other hand, maybe it was a clear and powerful calling.

Was your mom a doctor? Perhaps your grandfather was. Maybe there was a small-town pediatrician working countless hours out of his home. You know, the one who took care of you when you had a bad cough and, with a wink to you, told your mom to keep you home from school for a few days.

Was it TV's Dr. House seeing what nobody else could see, solving the impossible week after week, year after year, that turned you on to medicine? Maybe it was scenes on the TV news of doctors in multiple war-torn countries all over the world, helping victims of man's indecent acts against his fellow man, that grabbed your interest.

Who can forget how we watched countless doctors, from all over the world, rush to Haiti after the apocalyptic earthquake of 2010? What did they all have in common?

What is it that drives doctors day after day, week after week, and year after year to attend to the sick and needy? It is probably the very same thing that has motivated you to buy this book to help kick-start and improve your chances of getting into medical school.

Are you ready?

Let me ask you a question. Why *do* you want to be a doctor?

OK, let me hear it—the usual boring, automatic, humdrum response: "I want to be a doctor to help people."

Please. If I had a dollar for every time that I have heard this response, I seriously could have retired to my dream house in Italy years ago. If you want to help people, it is a lot easier, and much more lucrative, to be a plumber. I'm serious. Do the math. No college debt. No medical-school debt. Forget about the four-to-six years of residency and the malpractice insurance. Plumbers get $200 per hour for standard house calls, and that is just for showing up. Add to that the charge for your services. Then, if you mess up, they call you back to fix it, and you get to charge again for the new problem. And you don't get sued.

If you just want to help people, become a plumber. There will be more on this subject later in the book.

So are you still sure you want to go to medical school?

You know you have what it takes. You know that you work hard at it, especially compared to your friends who are just partying their way through life.

So what is it? How can you enhance your ability to get into medical school and actually make it happen? Notice that I didn't say "improve your chances"; I said "enhance your ability." We want to remove the word "chance" and make this a real improvement in ability. This is where you learn to be proactive and take charge of your life and future rather than be reactive and let others decide your fate.

Are you ready? Are you as excited as I am? Are you ready to take control of your future? Are you ready to start learning some of the insider information that will help you reach this goal? Are you ready to learn some of the secrets and tricks that will get you into medical school?

If you are, then let's get started. I will be your guide and your personal coach, training you for the "big event." But, as with every big event worth its salt, it will take a bit of work.

Let's get started.

1. Why a Doctor?

Here you are at your interview, elated and apprehensive at the same time. More than likely, you are alone. You are waiting to be directed to an office or meeting room for the big moment. Perhaps a group of applicants will be directed to the same place, and you realize that you are going to have a group interview (more on this in the chapter on interviews). You are unfazed. You are ready. You have prepared and know what you want to say and are reviewing your talking points in your head. You look around and see a group of very nervous, fidgety fellow applicants. Yet you remain calm. They look at you and completely don't understand your calmness. You have prepared.

You know that you are going to be asked lots of questions.

At this stage in the game, at the tail end of the medical-school application process, you sit back and reflect. You have worked hard. You have put in the time. You have spent countless hours in preparation. All you did prior to this day was really a process that got you to this time and place. All the work, all the preparation, was a way to get you noticed by an admissions-committee reviewer, who, after a meticulous review of your application, decided that you were the type of medical-school applicant who might be qualified and worthy of an interview.

Actually, the days of a single reviewer having the power to play God and decide single-handedly that you deserve an interview are over. The organizations that have oversight of the entire medical-school application process demand that medical schools have multiple application reviewers. This ensures a more democratic, fair medical-school application and review process.

You really have to come from a galaxy far, far away...

...if you don't anticipate being asked one particular question. If you haven't realized it by now, and I would certainly hope that you have, this is a question that you will not be able to out run, ignore, or hide from for the rest of your life. You will be asked at every party and social gathering you attend. You will be asked at ball games, PTA meetings, rock concerts, and restaurants.

They never stop asking.

Go ahead, have fun with it. Change your answer. Make up stuff. It doesn't matter, because most of the time, most people don't care. It's just a line, an icebreaker. It is a fill-in for when nobody knows what to say. They might as well be asking you, "What do you think about the weather?" By now you are probably thinking, *Hey, wait a minute, enough already. What's the question?* Well, I have been trying to avoid it. And you will try to avoid it, too, after you have been asked it a few thousand times. I am so tired of being asked this question at this stage in my life, and I try to avoid it as much as I can. But like I just said above, you, as an applicant and future doctor, just can't get away from it.

OK, OK, here it is, in your face. You asked for it. The question is, "Why do you want to be a doctor?"

You are going to be asked this question thousands of times over the next few decades. Other than your grandparents, most people are just making small talk, and they really could not care less. They may not even listen to the answer you decide to give them. All they hear is "Blah blah blah, and so on and so forth, and what have you." Or, as seen on TV: "Wa whomp, wa whomp, wa whomp." If you don't know what that last one was, go ask your parents; they'll know. (Hint: Charlie Brown in *Peanuts*.)

There is one great exception to the general ignoring public. When they ask you, "Why do you want to become a doctor?" they will be listening. What is this one exception? This will be at your interview and in your secondary application for medical school. Oops! I lied. That makes two exceptions. Believe me, they will listen and hang on to every word you say. They will grasp every nuance and inflection in your voice, body language, and the words that you pick.

On your application and at your medical-school interview, you had better answer this question succinctly and honestly. This question is a lot deeper than you might realize at first. This is actually a question that is multileveled and one from which an astute reviewer or interviewer will learn a great deal about you. You might be so smart that your immediate response may be, "I already wrote about that in my narrative, but I'll be happy to tell you again." I strongly urge you not to make that your answer. It will immediately label you as a wise guy and will turn off any interviewer. Just answer the question.

As I previously wrote, they already read about your childhood memories of your compassionate pediatrician, or how you learned to love medicine while working in a mission clinic on the Amazon River, or how the care (or lack of care) of a sick relative inspired you to become the most compassionate doctor in the whole universe.

They know you want to be a doctor by all of the lovely, motivational words that you compiled in your narratives in your primary and secondary applications. In spite of this, they will want to hear it in your own words and watch your body language as you answer the question.

The "Why do you want to be a doctor?" question is a very tricky question and one of my absolute favorites as an interviewer—not at any other time and not anywhere else. Yes, you read that right. I earlier said that I am so tired of being asked this question and try to avoid answering it these days. However, it is very different when you are sitting on the other side of the table and asking the question. As the interviewer, I (and any other interviewer) love to ask it. So my change of heart is due to the fact that I would be asking the question, not answering it.

The interviewer is waiting for you to give the usual, mundane, knee-jerk responses: "I love science, and becoming a doctor will give me the opportunity to use my scientific education in a fun, interesting way." Or, "I want to help the underserved." And then there is the most popular response of all...

"Because I want to help people in their time of greatest need and difficulty."

And they will let you go on and on about why you want to help people, especially in the time of their greatest need and difficulty. Hmm. The interviewers will then rub their chins, look at you pensively, and smile. They will look interested and appear as if they are hearing this response for the very first time.

Whew, you did it. You made it through that one. It went just the way you anticipated it would. You had practiced with your best friend, your advisor, your pet dog, and, God forbid, your parents. Of course, you practiced in front of your greatest fans, and they would never tell you anything other than exactly what you wanted to hear.

Another little digression. In the paraphrased words of Ross Perot, one of the most interesting Americans to ever have lived and the subject of Ken Follett's masterpiece novel, *On Wings of Eagles* (a novel that deals with the Iranian takeover of the American embassy in the late 1970s): "Surround yourself with advisors who will tell you what you *don't* want to hear." This is terrific advice and words that our national leaders should heed. This is one of the most important pieces of advice that I can offer to you in this book. History is full of examples of kings, queens, presidents, mayors, Indian chiefs, and so on, who surrounded themselves with advisors who just kissed up to them, resulting in disaster and tragedy.

OK. Getting back to the subject at hand...and then, with a smile, one of the interviewers says, "Well, how about I give you a call, say, at eleven o'clock at night, the next time my toilet backs up, overflows, and leaves me standing in *stuff*. And then that would be a time of 'great need and difficulty' for me. And besides, it would really be helping me." All of this is said with a smile.

What are you going to do? What can you say?

You just got finished saying that you want to help people, particularly during their time of greatest need and difficulty. So, do you politely give a little laugh and then clarify things a little? Perhaps you might say that you really want to help people during times of illness and infirmity. You might then be asked, "Well, why not become a nurse or physician's assistant?" Will you know how to answer that? Do you understand where this questioning is leading?

Think about it. Nurses and physicians' assistants clearly want to help people in their time of greatest need and difficulty. They are extremely well-educated and dedicated, and they live to serve and help. They see the sick and suffering. They see the ill and injured. They diagnose, and, in many settings, they can order appropriate medications and interventions. They are exactly who you are describing when you said that you want to help people, particularly during their time of greatest need and difficulty, and then tried to clarify this when you added that you really want to help people during times of illness and infirmity.

So, I ask you: "Why don't you become a nurse or physician's assistant?" They are two great professions that are full of well-educated, compassionate, giving, caring professionals who administer health care at the most skilled level.

How is this different from being a medical doctor?

What are you going to say?

You begin to panic. You can feel your heart pounding in your chest and desperately hope that your interviewer can't hear it. You are sweating. You practiced this one for weeks, over and over. In one fell swoop, your entire strategy for this question has been undermined.

You think hard. Your heart slows down. You begin to relax and allow yourself to settle in. There is a little flicker of understanding. A protean form begins to manifest itself at the outer most limits of your consciousness. It begins to coalesce. As it swirls and undulates through your conscious brain, a new thought begins to take form. You feel it coming as it slowly begins to ascend from the thought centers in your brain. Chemical reactions begin to intensify. Axons begin to light up. Impulses travel through neurons, and the message sparks across synapses. Finally, a clear thought congeals in your consciousness, and you realize that you have known the answer all along.

You focus and look the interviewer straight in the eye. The corners of your mouth lift up and form a knowing smile. You have it.

"As a physician, I assume responsibility."

The interviewer's eyes light up, still matching your stare; and then, slowly and knowingly, he/she nods with a smile. There is an approving nod to your response.

When you are a physician, you assume the mantle of captain of the ship. Ultimate responsibility is yours and only yours. If you are in a group practice, hospital or clinic-based practice, solo private practice, or on a medical mission, you are in charge. The responsibility is yours. In the immortal, paraphrased words of our thirty-sixth president, Harry Truman, the buck stops with you. In actuality, when he was president, Harry Truman had a sign on his desk that faced out for anyone sitting across from him to see. It said: "The Buck Stops Here!"

You are responsible.

This is what sets you apart. Responsibility. It is the acceptance of being the ultimate decision maker and being culpable for your decisions, which are the ultimate responsibilities and obligations you take on when you sign on to become a doctor.

This is what you have signed up for. So be very clear on this one.

My intention is not to state anything that is politically incorrect. There are more than a few instances when nurses and other members of the allied medical professions carry great responsibilities and make life-changing decisions; and in almost every situation, they are supervised by and responsible to a senior physician. But every physician is the captain of his or her own ship, at all times—24-7! Please be clear that I have met, and know, many physicians' assistants ("assistant" is built into the name), nurses, medical assistants, and technicians who are infinitely smarter and more intuitive than a great many of the physicians I have met. My mission is not to impugn their integrity (legalese) or denigrate them in any way. My mission is to help you and guide you to truly dig deep into yourself. My goal is to help you fully understand what you are all about.

On first blush it is so easy to answer the question when you are asked, "Why do you want to be a doctor?" Most doctors and medical-school applicants immediately answer, "I want to help people." It's easy to say because that is what you really want to do. Now you are beginning to understand what it is that sets you apart from others in the health-care profession. You might not have consciously known or understood it before. It is just a part of your natural makeup. It is the responsibility, the leadership, and the decision making that comes with it that you are searching for. It is this role that you are craving. It is no simple thing.

Not everybody has what it takes to become a doctor. Not everybody is willing to make the tremendously difficult decisions that are required on a daily basis. Heck, did I say daily? Well, how about on a minute-to-minute basis? For trauma specialists, cardiologists, intensivists, and *every* intern and resident, it is a constant reality. It is their daily lives and is inherent to who they truly are. It makes their blood flow and is part of their DNA. These incredible men and women often have multiple critical, life-threatening scenarios unfolding and playing out simultaneously. They must make decisions, take responsibility, delegate appropriately, and focus (refer to the chapter titled "Focus"). They take ultimate responsibility for every patient that they have treated, are treating, or are about to treat.

When you are accepted to medical school, it is the first in a series of huge steps. Your life is on the verge of change—a very radical change. You are being given the opportunity to open and enter through a door that will be the portal to an amazing new world. It is a world of magic, a world of unveiled secrets. It is world in which science, ethics, and metaphysics will pull at you or come to your aid to enable you to weave your way through the continuous stream of challenges that you will encounter from the moment you step through the entryway.

What you will learn in medical school—physiology, microbiology, genetics, ethics, professionalism, renal endocrinology, cardiology, pediatrics, medical clerkships, surgical clerkships, internship, residency—all of it is designed to prepare you to become a new doctor who is ready to totally take on this very special mantle of responsibility. It is a serious, awesome responsibility of biblical proportions. I am not speaking with hyperbole.

You will be making decisions and hold the responsibility that will decide the fate—life or death—of your fellow human beings.

Everyone in medicine—the laboratory technician, the medical assistant, the aide, the nurse, the physician's assistant, and the physician—has responsibilities. They all are responsible and have received this mantle with the complete understanding of what they have dedicated themselves to.

Please remember what sets you apart. Please never forget. Please never lose the fire, passion, focus, and compassion. You have accepted the ultimate responsibility. All of the others have someone else to turn to, someone to guide them, to offer suggestions, or to take over if the going gets a little too tough. They have someone else to bail them out if they need it. They have someone else to tell them that they need assistance, guidance, or replacement if they don't see it for themselves.

You are the doctor. You are the one who brings congratulations to new parents. It is you who will bring good news to an ailing patient. You are the one who gets to place a hand on a shoulder for reassurance to a husband or wife. Of course, all other allied health and medical professionals want to do these things, too. In truth, they do get to do these wonderful, heartwarming tasks, probably just not as often as you will get to.

But rest assured, you, the doctor, have an additional task. You also get to assume and accept what the others are not willing to assume or accept. You get to walk along a difficult, hazardous path. At each fork along this trail, you will accept that you will always have to choose the more demanding path. You will have the onerous task and the responsibility of telling the bad news, rendering the heartbreak, being the minion of the destruction of dreams, and being the messenger delivering the word of loss of loved ones. You are the messenger who turns a life or a world upside down. You will be there, and should be there, to offer a shoulder and your understanding. You are there to ease the pain and suffering.

You are the doctor. You are *their* doctor. You are their yin and yang. One day you may be my doctor (and please be sure to let me know that you have read this book).

Getting back to where we started: You are at your interview. Everything is going smoothly. You are coasting. You have gotten through the tougher questions (please see chapter 18). You think that you are home free. The interviewers sit back and fold their arms, and small smiles cross their lips. Then one of them very smoothly removes his or her glasses. The interviewer unwaveringly looks directly and deeply into your eyes. You sense lips moving, and you don't even have to hear the words that you have been waiting for and anticipating for the past thirty minutes. And then the interviewer asks you, "Why do you want to be a doctor?"

Now you know what they are really asking. You understand that they are looking for certain qualities. They are looking for passion, dedication, focus, compassion, and leadership. With this question, they are really searching for your understanding that you are dedicating yourself to assuming the ultimate mantle of responsibility that our society of human beings is willing to bestow upon you as a fellow human being, and you are 100 percent willing to accept.

You are taking on the ultimate responsibility of answering questions and making decisions that will have a tremendous impact on the health, welfare, and quality of life of your fellow human beings. And very likely you will be making decisions that ultimately decide between life and death.

This huge responsibility is staggering. Most who are in a position to decide will turn away to pursue easier paths. Most will not and cannot even consider carrying such a weight on their shoulders. It is up to you to decide if it is a wonderful gift or a horrible burden. Almost all who enter into this noble profession see it as a gift and privilege. So now I sit back and fold my arms; a small smile crosses my lips;

and then, very smoothly, I remove my glasses. I look unwaveringly directly and deeply into your eyes. You are aware that my lips are moving, and you don't even have to hear the words that you have been anticipating for the past thirty minutes. Let me ask you...

"Why do you want to be a doctor?"

2. Focus

Let's go back to August 2005. Hurricane Katrina was sitting on top of New Orleans. Being a category 5 hurricane with top winds in the range of 170 miles per hour, Katrina brought destruction, misery, and sorrow to New Orleans and her people. As I write this book today, almost a decade later, New Orleans still hasn't completely recovered. Reconstruction continues, and the city is once again beginning to thrive.

Now let's time-travel to 2009. The New Orleans Saints had never even made it through the playoffs, let alone to the Super Bowl. But this year was different. There was a change. It was almost as if the Saints were group-hypnotized. There was a charge in the atmosphere surrounding New Orleans. The 2009 Saints were shepherded with inscrutable, unswerving craftsmanship. They were led by a powerful force—a force by the name of Drew Brees, their quarterback. The Saints were a team that had never made it through the long postseason playoffs. And then in 2009, it happened. The long drought was over. They did it. The New Orleans Saints won their first National Football Conference (NFC). The electricity continued to flow, and then they went on to win Super Bowl XLIV, their one and only Super Bowl. This seemingly miraculous event occurred a mere four years after Hurricane Katrina devastated New Orleans and their home stadium. How did this miracle happen?

Just months earlier, the "drama on the Hudson" had unfolded. It was a clear, beautiful day in New York City. The roads, waterways, and skies surrounding New York City were uncongested, and all was business as usual. US Airways Flight 1549 was cleared for takeoff and taxied down the auxiliary runway, turned onto the main runway, revved her engines, and then ascended. Six minutes after takeoff from New York's LaGuardia Airport, nature intervened. A phalanx of Canadian geese was in the flight path. Collision between the engines and the geese was unavoidable, and the engines were disabled. Just as nature had intervened, so did providence. It just so happened that the senior pilot of this flight was seasoned and experienced. Captain Chesley "Sully" Sullenberger coolly and calmly commanded his jet and crew. He performed the necessary maneuvers to avoid catastrophe and guided US 1549 to a safe water landing on the frigid Hudson River. He saved the lives of all 155 people on his aircraft.

In 1996, the world was engrossed with the events that unfolded atop the 29,029 foot peak of Mount Everest. A few years later, the tragic and heroic events were beautifully chronicled in the riveting bestselling book *Into Thin Air* by John Krakauer. In the mid-1990s, the ascent of Mount Everest had become an adventure-tourist Mecca. The wealthy and adventurous had incorporated this feat into their personal bucket lists. Since Sir Edmund Hilliary and Sherpa Tenzing Norgay first summited Everest in 1953, it had remained in the domain of professional mountain climbers. But with the advent of adventure travel marketing and the development of affordable technology for climbing, the summit was reachable for those who could afford the staggering $65,000 (1996) fee. The rampant inexperience and lack of professionalism predicted the disaster that was to come for an expedition to the top. After a series of amateur mistakes and a "rogue" storm, eight of the climbers of two expeditions perished from exposure on Mount Everest, including two of the leading mountain guides in the world. The rescue team was led by America's premier "Everest climber" Peter Athans, who lived in Boulder, Colorado, and lived the life of a professional mountaineer. His life was spent planning and leading mountain expeditions. It was Peter Athans, who happened to be in the Himalayas at the time of the Everest disaster, who was asked to lead the heroic emergency expedition that successfully saved the lives of the remaining climbers. Athans's success can be attributed to his decades of mountaineering experience and his professionalism.

What do these heroes have in common? What does this have to do with you getting into medical school? What does this have to do with this book?

These people were, and are, focused throughout all of their years of education and training. They remained focused throughout all of their years of active participation in the pursuit of their individual passions. They were focused during these life-defining episodes where they accomplished their superhuman achievements. They were focused in every aspect of their lives. Focus was the great enabler that gave them the ability to accomplish their goals or missions.

Would you like to have this brand of focus? You can, and you will!

Look around you. Who are your heroes? Who are the giants, the most successful people in our society? Whom do we see on TV and in newspapers who are there for positive reasons? Who are these people? What makes them famous and as successful as they are? Why do we want to be like them? Why do we aspire to have the qualities that they have? Well, let me ask you: What is the singular characteristic that they all have in common?

They are focused!

I have just recounted for you three extraordinary stories of three extraordinary humans. They are heroes and professionals, but they also have real lives and know how to have fun. During the events just related, they were focused, always focused.

In order to achieve a goal, any goal, you must be focused.

Becoming a doctor—not just getting into medical school but becoming the best doctor that you can be—will require this same level of focus that I have just described to you above. You can do it too. You can achieve what these three intrepid professionals achieved. In fact, anyone can do it.

If you already have it, you know it. If not, I can guarantee to you that if you read and absorb all that I will reveal to you in this book and earnestly follow my suggestions, you will automatically develop the focus that will enable you to pursue your dream of becoming a doctor. Or for that matter, any other dream that is your passion.

You are at home and sitting at your desk studying. You have just finished a totally frustrating, incomprehensible forty-five minutes of organic chemistry review. You sit back and ask yourself, "What did I just spend the last forty-five minutes of my life doing?" You still have assignments in psychology and physics to complete. Papers are everywhere, and books are piled up in front of you, teetering in front of you like a mad professor. The big homecoming game is tomorrow, and you really want to go because you were told that the hottie who sits across the aisle from you in class will be there. Argh, you just can't focus.

And then the phone rings, interrupting your downward spiral. It's your best friend inviting you to meet up with a bunch of friends at the local sports bar. "Let's go out and have some fun. Let's chill."

This is it, the break, the lifeline that you have been waiting for—the excuse to run away from your desk, the frustration, and the difficulty. After all, what are friends for? Do you go for it? The answer, in a word, is no. You have to stay focused.

First of all, you should have had a long-term study plan (more on this in a later chapter) to facilitate the utilization of your already deficient time that would have given you the added bonus of less frustration and confusion. But let's get back to the issue at hand. This is a decisive moment. If you had planned to go out with your friends to party or relax or shop or fold origami, that would be fine. You would have had an incentive, a gift to reward yourself with after you had completed your hard, organized studies. But in this situation, it is an excuse to drop the ball and run, with almost certainly disastrous results.

All of this mess resulted from the simple lack of focus.

How do we develop focus?

Some of us learned this skill as a child. Just a few decades ago, I spent many afternoons building model airplanes and ships while my friends were out getting into trouble. Today I love to watch the undeterred focus of my fifteen-year-old son as he destroys an imaginary enemy in *Modern Warfare* on his Xbox. Now this is total focus. Equally thrilling is to observe my thirteen-year-old daughter as she controls her environment as an infielder on her fast-pitch softball team. They are both honing their respective focusing skills. This is a tool that will serve them the rest of their lives.

Yes, it's a tool that will serve them—and serve you the rest of your life, too. Focus.

So, if you haven't excelled in Xbox or fast-pitch softball, are you lost? Game over?

Nah!

There are so many ways to learn to be focused. Yoga, meditation, Tai Chi, and chess are wonderful, relaxing ways to develop your focusing skills.

Here's a thought. Why do you think so many thousands of people play golf? Sure it's fun, but there is a whole additional dimension to it. When you play golf, you automatically tune out all the other stuff in your busy day, and you focus. Most golfers even turn off their cell phones while on the golf course and look scornfully at others who don't. Then as a bonus, as you play the game over weeks and months, your focus improves. This is one of the main reasons successful people tend to be good golfers.

If golf isn't for you, there is running, sailing, tennis, rock climbing (lots of indoor facilities), cerebral computer games, and the list goes on. There are so many ways to develop focus.

Unlike dieters, don't start tomorrow. Dieters are always starting tomorrow. They are the same people that are always putting things off, procrastinating. In fact, there is a billion-dollar industry built around this form of procrastination. Please be assured, I am not judging anyone's physical fitness. I am only referring to the "diet" mentality.

I suggest you start today.

Here is an exercise that you can do to help you learn how to focus. Sit down on a comfortable chair or sofa. Look straight ahead and pick a spot, any spot, and stare at it. Don't gaze away from the spot. Stay on that spot. Don't divert your gaze away from the spot. Don't look at anything else. And please don't do this while you are driving!

Take in some nice slow, deep breaths through your nose. Exhale slowly through your nose. Repeat this three times. As you continue to stare at your point, close your eyes slowly. Look through your eyelids at your point. Visualize it and see it through your closed eyelids. Deepen your breathing and slow it down. Count with each inhalation. One, two, three...up to ten, all the while visualizing your point. Now, let this point expand, slowly growing and radiating out. As it expands, allow it to emit light. You will feel the energy and be invigorated. Stay with it. Absorb it. Focus on it. You will know intuitively when it is time to release it. Then, as you continue to breathe slowly and deeply, count back ten, nine...to one. Slowly open your eyes.

This is your first lesson in learning to focus.

Believe me, as you practice this exercise, once or twice each day, it will become easier and more comfortable. A good time to practice this focus exercise is when you are multitasking or feeling stressed and overwhelmed. When the noise of life clutters your mind, stop and journey to your point. It will take time and work to develop this tool, but all good things take time and work. Practice, practice, practice. But it won't take you to Carnegie Hall. (A very old joke. Sorry.) So please do work on this. After all, it is going to take time and hard work for you to get into medical school and develop into the best doctor that you can be.

Interestingly, as we learn to master our focus, we learn to easily tune out all of the extraneous noise in our lives. "Did I turn off the bathtub?" "Gee, I want a date with (you can fill in the blank)." "I can't wait to tell so-and-so about so-and-so." "I hope I can beat the traffic home tonight." And the list can go on and on. You get the gist of it.

There is so much noise out there. The day is full of distractions. Some are good, and some are really annoying. But to reach your goal, any goal, you must focus. It is a major part of our lives as doctors. With time, patience, and plenty of practice, you will become good at it.

In fact, a very strong factor as to which medical specialty that one will choose is based on their ability to focus. If you are truly OCD (have obsessive-compulsive disorder) and have an uncanny ability to focus, you might consider microsurgery or craniofacial surgery. There are other specialties that don't require as much OCD focus, but believe me, every doctor has developed a highly refined ability to focus. This is what enables doctors to excel at what they do. It is this focus and high demand for excellence that makes American medicine the best in the world.

This is not a comment on American health-care delivery and the ever-increasing difficulties being faced in the United States in the implementation and distribution of health care. I am simply stating that the training, technology, and application of medicine in the United States is the best in the world.

As we become better at focusing, we don't have to worry about all of the other, less important items that can clutter our minds and time. Or, as the popular expression so simply states, we learn "not to sweat the small stuff."

So, how does one tune out the noise and clatter?

A simple, effective tool used to concentrate on the task at hand and sharpen your focus is one that many highly successful people utilize when they are faced with overwhelming projects and tasks. It is also highly effective when one is faced with numerous sequential or simultaneous tasks.

If you are someone who is easily daunted by these types of situations, or you have become the master procrastinator, then this tool will work particularly well for you.

You will see *immediate results* the first time you decide to apply this simple technique. In fact, you probably have already mastered it without realizing it. Almost all students have. You might call it "cramming."

Yes, that's right. I am advocating cramming as an effective way to develop and perfect your innate ability to focus and succeed. But we are going to tweak it a little and cheat a little, too. Instead of cramming the night before an exam or before the big assignment is due, you are going to cram every day or night, day after day, week after week, month after month. You get the picture, right?

You see, by setting—and religiously adhering to—a predetermined amount of study time each day, you create an artificial environment of stress, with the release of internal catecholamine (adrenaline) and small amounts of cortisol (stress hormone that your adrenal glands produce).

The way you do it is to decide in advance how much time you are going study each day for a given period of time. For example, you set it up so that you will have exactly two hours to study every evening for the next two weeks. No more, no less. You must stick to the time parameters without failure and without any departures. You must find work to fill the two hours. But you cannot exceed the two hours on any given day. If two hours isn't realistic for you, then set the time parameter for a realistic goal for *you*. You will find that this sets up efficient utilization of time and forces you to focus. In addition, by underestimating the time, you create positive stress with release of catecholamine and cortisol. These two hormones will then work together to improve your speed of covering your materials, increase your understanding, augment your assimilation, boost your recall, and enhance the application of your newfound information.

You will produce an environment of inducing "good stress," which is a human adaptation for production and excellence. You will also halt the manifestation of destructive, life-shortening, and disease-producing "bad stress" by adhering to this daily routine.

You see, by knowing that you have a limited amount of time to complete your task(s), your mind enters a state of hyper-efficiency, which increases your memory, analytical skills, assimilation of concepts, and application of concepts. By doing this day in and day out, you will be absolutely amazed with what you will be able to accomplish.

So there you have it. I have shared with you a couple of very effective, powerful tools that will enable you, immediately, to sharpen your focus and zoom in on your dreams.

Focus is one of the life tools that will enhance your ability, in so many ways, to become a top-notch medical-school applicant. Focus is a life tool that will enhance your ability to become a terrific doctor. Focus is a life tool that will enable you to become the best human being that you can become and improve the quality of life for you, your loved ones, your patients, and your community.

3. Certainty

Once again, I would like to call your attention to a trait that highly successful people seemingly always demonstrate. Nope, not focus, but a trait that is far more subtle.

Some people are born with it. Some have it developed, nurtured, and trained into them by loving, knowledgeable parents. Other people are lucky enough to be exposed to it and begin to catch a glimmer of it later in their lives.

Once anyone gets a taste of it, it's all over for him or her because it becomes addictive.

It defines a way of life and is very fulfilling. It is a force so powerful that when utilized appropriately, it practically guarantees success in almost any endeavor or challenge that exists.

Michael Jordan was a master. Do you think that he ever thought about missing a shot to the basket? What about the famous multiple Olympic gold champion of speed skating, Apolo Ohno? He only talked about winning, and win he did. Sir Edmund Hillary, the first to summit Mount Everest, let everyone know that he was going to succeed where all others before him had failed. He lived and breathed the summit.

Tiger Woods was among this august group, but he let it slip away. Why did he become second best, twentieth best, and frequently an "also ran"?

He forgot the secret.

What do you think is the secret behind how these famous exemplars were able to achieve what they did, become what they are, change a course of events or history, and create an ever-enduring legacy?

Yes, they have all worked hard to achieve what they accomplished and demonstrated complete dedication. But we all work hard for our achievements, especially students who want to get into medical school.

So what is it that sets these "super people" apart?

In a word, *certainty*.

Certainty. The ultimate form of visualization.

Or, perhaps better said in today's lexicon, "extreme visualization."

How does it begin? Where does it come from? What is the source? Actually, the answer is pretty simple and clear-cut. It all starts with a thought. That's right, a simple thought!

At first it might be subconscious; a subconscious thought that is not even perceived by the conscious side of your brain. A series of chemical reactions are initiated by something that you may have heard or seen—for example, friends speaking, a television show, or a movie.

Maybe a friend suggested that you read this book, or it was suggested to you on the Internet, and you really didn't pay the particular suggestion any heed. It was in your subconscious. But, the seed was planted. The seed was planted somewhere deep in that part of your brain that is the incubator for your thoughts. More than likely you weren't even receptive to this fortuitous encounter.

Well, my friend, the seed was planted, and like all seeds all around the world, once a seed is planted, it has two pathways. Paraphrasing the great Bard with a little linguistic license: To grow or not to grow, that is the question. Whether or not to suffer the slings and arrows of outrageous fortune. And so on, and so forth.

As you have already learned earlier in this book, you are not going to succumb to outrageous fortune; you will be proactive and take charge.

As I was saying, "To grow or not to grow." Your seed has been planted in a fertile environment that is rich with nutrients, oxygen, and fertilizer. Yup, there is some BS (bodacious stuff) up there fertilizing your brain.

So one day you are lying out in a beautiful grassy field. You know, that incredibly green field somewhere in Kansas that is pictured on so many Microsoft wallpapers. Big, puffy cumulus clouds slowly float above, like a flock of sheep endlessly grazing in the great blue. All is well in your life. There is no blocking noise or chaos in your life. The environment is perfect in your brain. As you lie there, your brain has become a primordial medium without blockages or interferences.

And so your seed begins to germinate, and sprout, send out roots, and grow, and become...wait for it...boiiiiinggg...a thought!

The subconscious seed has become a conscious thought.

It has broken through the surface and, at long last, has appeared on your personal radar. It is still yours and only yours. It is floating there in your primordial soup, waiting. What happens next? Your cell phone rings! The thought disappears, withers away—gone. It sinks to the sediment at the bottom of the soup. But it's not gone forever. It waits for you. It will be back. All you have to do is open a window, and whoosh, it is back.

You might ask, "How do I do that? How can I retrieve it if it isn't even a conscious thought?"

As it is no longer floating just below the surface of your consciousness, it has sunk back down to the bottom sediment. How do you bring it back? The answer is really quite simple.

Don't think about anything!

Get rid of your cell phone, iPad, iPhone, TV, and all of the other distractors.

Give yourself a break. Take ten to fifteen minutes every day to think. Think about nothing. That's right, take ten to fifteen minutes every day to clear your mind, to remove the noise, and to eliminate the chaos that is tangling it all up.

You also need to remove the analytical, the objective, and the cognizant thoughts that have held your mind hostage for many years. You need ten to fifteen minutes daily to let the seeds germinate and grow and to come to the surface. You must allow the seeds to ascend, to float, to sprout, to establish roots, to spread, and to grow.

Once the seed resurfaces and roots are allowed to establish themselves, the thought will gain stability and then have the ability to enter the realm of your conscious mind.

You have prepared yourself and given yourself permission to receive and process this previously subconscious nugget in the conscious part of your brain. The thought is able to enter that part of your consciousness that will allow you to ponder and play with it; to roll it around; and to stretch, shrink, expand, and morph it in any way you see fit.

This thought is your own. In your personal domain, you are in charge. Have fun with it in any way that you wish.

Look at it from the front, the back, the top, the bottom, and each side. Step into it and see the world from the viewpoint of your new thought. Maybe you can look at the world from the peak of this new mountaintop—this pinnacle of new thought. I'll bet you that the whole world will look a little different to you when you look at it from this new vantage point.

My point is that with your new thought, the one created from the protean soup of chemicals, electrical impulses, random amalgamations, and connections in your brain, you can change the whole world. At the very least, you will change your personal world and all those whom you come into contact with.

If you think it, it will be.

Plato did it. So did Newton, Shakespeare, and Mother Teresa. So enjoy the ride, the roller coaster of freeing your mind and allowing all sorts of fun ideas to pop in.

This is a very powerful tool for you to utilize in almost every step of your pursuit of becoming a doctor. You will be regularly challenged with what might appear to be insurmountable challenges and barraged with multiple little crazy nuisances and irritations. Each challenge in life and each blockage is an opportunity for you to grow, to improve, and to become better as you move forward toward your ultimate goal.

Don't let these challenges and blockages in life frustrate you or stop you in your quest. See these events for what they truly are: opportunities for growth and advancement.

I am sure that you must know people, perhaps friends or acquaintances, who just always seem to land on their feet. No matter what challenges they face, no matter what roadblocks are set in their path, they just seem to always come through it and usually are all the better for the experience.

You certainly must know people like that. They are always successful and seem to be always basking in the glow. They are the ones who always manage to turn lemons into lemonade. They turn chicken s--t into chicken salad.

This is the whole point of this chapter. If you think it, it will be. But you must think it with certainty.

Just like Michael Jordan, Apolo Ohno, and Sir Edmund Hillary, whom I wrote about at the beginning of this chapter, nothing is going to stop you.

What is the common theme here?

It is all about certainty.

If you think it, it will be. Always.

Rhonda Byrne made millions of dollars by using her positivity to affect millions of people and change their lives forever. The theme of her best-selling book *The Secret* was that certainty with which you can achieve just about anything.

By putting the message of certainty out there to the universe with total belief and conviction, you can achieve, receive, create, conjure, conquer, build, and accomplish anything.

With certainty, you can accomplish anything!

You only have to experience it once, perhaps twice, to be convinced and believe it. Those of us who have been there a few times are ardent believers and live by it.

I remember the first time I submitted an abstract for the presentation of some of my original clinical research for a National Medical Specialty Society meeting. Acceptance of an abstract, after review, almost guaranteed publication in the specialty's peer-reviewed journal. At that time, I had already published quite a few peer-reviewed articles and case reports in well-respected medical journals. But this was my first piece on primary clinical research.

I thought it was earthshaking new information and felt that it *had to be* published. Well, as you have already guessed, it was summarily, and not so kindly, rejected. Wow, what a blow to my ego. But I knew that it had to be published.

So I emptied my brain and let go of all conscious thought. The juices flowed, the synapses sparked, connections, disconnections, reconnections...and then—boiiiiinggg—a brand-new thought surfaced. A seed was planted and germinated and established its roots. I reanalyzed my data, and lo and behold, there was much deeper and better stuff. Stuff of greater significance; stuff that I just had to write down and disseminate to my colleagues. Well, you guessed the outcome. The revised, improved abstract was approved and accepted. I presented my research, and it was published. It became one of the most cited journal articles on the subject in medical literature. To this day I still receive communications from my colleagues about this work.

When you empty your brain of thought and eliminate the clatter, the subconscious seeds arise and germinate into new conscious thoughts.

So now you can see how the process works. An open, clear mind, combined with certainty, is a powerful tool. These are tools that you can develop and utilize, take advantage of in your quest to get into medical school and design your future—an amazing future of being the best doctor that you can be.

Let's get back to the original point of this discussion. I do tend to go off on tangents (a slight understatement). It is just the way I think, the way my mind works. In fact, many people think and express themselves in this way. It takes a little work to communicate your thoughts in an organized fashion. But this is the whole point of the above discussion.

Just let the thoughts create themselves; let them percolate; let them rise from the abyss and work their way to the surface of your consciousness. Worry about organizing them afterward. Anyone can be an organizer. But how many people out there can come up with original thoughts and ideas on a regular basis?

Your brain is organized (pun intended) in such a manner as to allow you to perform several tasks at once, in addition to controlling your heartbeat, respiration, and all of the other thousands of basic functions of life. If you have the gift of being able to allow new, creative thoughts to arise while simultaneously doing what your conscious mind requires, then you are a step ahead of most people.

My generation was trained and schooled in an era when "silence" was considered "golden." No distractions were to be had while studying. We were brainwashed and conditioned to study in soundproof libraries, study halls, or, if you had the luxury, a very quiet bedroom at home.

This myth of the need for absolute silence to facilitate learning or creativity has been perpetuated for centuries.

Today we live in a different world. Sound waves are everywhere. Visual distractions abound. My kids have been studying with the computer on; the television sending out a steady stream of noise; iPods, iPads, and iPhones all on. Add to that the simultaneous playing of *Call of Duty*, *Grand Theft Auto*, and *Minecraft*. Now throw in Xbox Live. Yet, with all of this sensory overload, they have been pulling off straight A's.

I have learned to become flexible, and like many generations before me, I have come to accept the changing dynamic of our society. That is, as long as my kids keep getting their straight A's.

Finally, getting back to certainty. Our discussion now takes us to the question of mind over matter. Tony Robbins includes this as a major point in his motivational seminars in positive thinking. He invites and encourages his audience participants to walk on hot coals. The audience participants complete the task without feeling pain or suffering from any burns.

Dr. Masuro Emoto has demonstrated the process of how positive, and negative, thoughts of an observer directly influence the growth and shape of ice crystals. His studies are startling and easily accessible on the Internet.

Today you can see for yourself a clear and easily understandable demonstration of mind over matter. In fact, you can see it clearly demonstrated right now at any one of the numerous hands-on children's museums across the country. This oracular mind-over-matter apparatus is fascinating and a lot of fun to play with alone, with kids, or with friends. My son (twelve at the time) and my daughter (ten at the time) totally blew me away, destroyed me. Of course, I can use the excuse that they have had many hours of training by playing Xbox and Wii. I know, I know, that's a pretty lame excuse. They slaughtered me because children are inherently much more accepting of change and are much less orthodox in their thinking.

For children, things don't always have to make sense. Children are more accepting and receptive to what is occurring in front of them without the adult need for interpretation.

Here is how the game works. You sit at a table that has a little electrostatically charged ball sitting in a track on a table. You put on a small headset that contains microreceivers that will pick up your brain waves. Not that much different than the electrodes of an EEG (electroencephalogram) but without the needles to pierce the skin. The headset is wired to the track upon which the ball rests. You then sit there and stare at the ball. You are supposed to move the ball down the track, away from you, solely by the strength of your will and determination.

Based upon your level of concentration, the ball will either move forward or backward. All the while, your opponent is doing the same thing from across the table. Here's the kicker. The track is wired so that the ball moves forward only when you think calm thoughts. The more you think of moving the ball forward, the more backward the ball moves. I guess you can really say that this is an example of "mind over antimatter." Just a joke.

Your mind (brain waves) is in total control of matter (the ball).

This is just an example of science catching up to what many people have known throughout the ages. Mind over matter has been around for a very, very long time. How about this?

How many times in your lifetime have you, out of nowhere, started to think about someone—a friend, a colleague, or a loved one whom you haven't seen or heard from in a long time? Someone you haven't even thought about in a hugely long time—I'm talking months or years. For no reason at all, out of the clear blue, you start thinking about this person. Then suddenly he or she appears—at a restaurant or at the mall or at a party or in a car next to you at the only traffic light in a small farm town on a country road in the middle of nowhere.

This actually happened to me just a few weeks prior to starting the writing of this book. It involved a close friend whom I hadn't seen or spoken with in months. She was returning from a triathlon on the other side of the state. She had some life issues, and she needed help in resolving them. She had been thinking of me and how I would be able to help her. She really needed my help and was thinking intensely of getting in touch with me.

I had been thinking of her a lot over several days. I was returning home after spending a few days at a beautiful beach resort. Over the past year, I had wanted to take her to this beautiful tropical paradise and never had the opportunity. During my entire stay there, I had been thinking of her.

There I was, literally driving across the state. I was geographically right in the middle of the state, and again I was thinking about her, intensely. And then, "poof," there we both were, sitting in our cars, stopped at the only traffic light in a small farm town in the middle of nowhere. It shocked both of us, and the incident irrevocably strengthened our wonderful friendship. Coincidence? I think not!

This was a strong demonstration of mind over matter. Two minds were thinking about each other, intensely. Both minds sent out waves, needing the connection. The signals were sent out. There was an interplay of electrical activity. There was a reaction.

To make this story a little more interesting, I was driving back home on the very same day that I had just visited the interactive children's science museum that had the electrostatically charged ball headset apparatus example of mind over matter. Wow! You can imagine what kind of day that was.

Part and parcel to this discussion of certainty...Part and parcel? What the heck does that really mean? We all use this expression without giving it any thought. A part of what? A parcel of what? What a crazy expression. It doesn't have any meaning. Really, now. Actually, it is an American bastardization of the nobler Latin *pari passu*, which means "on equal footing." Sorry about the digression. Just a pet peeve. Pet peeve? What the heck is a pet peeve? Oh, never mind.

So, pari passu to this discussion of certainty, I feel obligated to introduce you to the field of noetic science. This is a field that was pioneered by Apollo 15 astronaut Edgar Mitchell when he returned to Earth. He expressed that the earth was part of a living system and that we all live "in a universe of consciousness." This is an example of the current growing cultural phenomenon in the belief of global consciousness. George Lucas also made his grand statement on the topic in the movie *Avatar*. I strongly recommend that you see it.

As you develop your ability to conceive and grow new thoughts, please don't let them be just new thoughts. Remember to ponder, muddle, flip, rotate, and dwell. Then, when they are clear and have a definitive purpose, act upon them with certainty.

Make your dream(s) your reality.

4. Glass Half Full?

You sit there, alone—all alone in a vast emptiness.

You sit in a cold, empty space. There is a rock-hard protuberance jabbing you in your lower back, causing your lower ribs to ache. You suddenly realize that you are strapped by your arms and legs to a hard, wooden stiff-backed chair. You are feeling isolated and wondering what is to come.

Then you look again at "it." There it is right before you: a solid black, homogenous, depthless, ominous background. It is infinite, stretching on endlessly. Then pain erupts in your eyes in a flash. On bursts a highly focused halogen spotlight, which brightly illuminates an object that seems to be floating in air. But then you realize that it is sitting on a pedestal draped in black, which melts into the black infinity surrounding it.

The intense light starkly highlights the transparency of the solitary tall glass.

One might say that this tall glass is half empty.

An invisible voice drones on. It surrounds you and echoes through the chamber and makes your ears vibrate. It feels like it passes through your head. It asks you the same question again and again.

"What do you see?"

Over and over you give the same response: "I see a half-empty glass." You are tired, stressed, and afraid. You plead, "What do they want me to say?" You think hard and deep within. Finally, in a desperate attempt, and with overzealous self-satisfaction, you erupt with "I see a glass that is half full!"

You know that you nailed it. You will be released. You will be able to move on. You will be free. The great stress abates. The fear has resolved.

Unfortunately, this is how too many medical-school applicants feel at their interview—imprisoned in an unearthly environment.

Getting back to our story: You feel that you have successfully found the key to your freedom. You have answered the question correctly. You think that you have given them what they want. The lights come on. The restraining straps autorelease. You are free to move on. Hardly!

You have fallen into the "mediocrity trap." You didn't really think about your response. You gave them what you thought they wanted to hear, or worse, you regurgitated a memorized response.

Mediocrity will not set you above the rest. It will not set you in front of the masses. You will not be a standout.

You need to be *the standout.*

When I speak to premedical and preprofessional groups of students, I love to bring up this point. I don't turn out the lights, strap them down, or sensory deprive them. But I present them with a beautiful photograph of a tumbler that is half empty or half full. When I ask them what they see, their responses are as you would imagine.

A few of the students will state that they see a glass that is half empty. And then there is the larger group that boastfully shouts out that they see a glass that is half full. And then, as I always do at this point, I smile and slowly shake my head sideways in a paternal way to indicate no.

You see, we have all learned conditioned responses. In life there will be many opportunities for you to be challenged with questions as to your perceptions of a particular observation or scenario.

To achieve your desired goal in the particular circumstance you are faced with—an essay, a presentation, a medical-school interview, a postgraduate residency interview—you must change your mentality.

To give the expected correct, conditioned response is a surefire way to be lost in the masses. But if you give a well-thought-out, extraordinary (literally *extra ordinary*) response, it will set you well above and ahead of everyone else.

Let's get back to that half-empty/half-full glass of water. As I have already related to you, the so-called glass-is-half-full perspective is the "new way of thinking" conditioned response. You might even say it is a modern point of view. That is anything but the truth. It is a boring, thoughtless answer. It is mediocrity personified. You don't want to be mediocre. You want to be, and need to be, a standout.

When you see that half-empty/half-full glass of water, why not look at it in an inspired and in an extraordinary way? Why not use the new way of thinking that I have been working so hard to teach you throughout this book?

When you see a glass with water in it, you just might consider responding by stating exactly what you see.

How about responding by saying, "I see a glass with water in it." And then if you really get into it, you might say, "I see a way to give comfort to the thirsty." "I see a way to hydrate the dehydrated." "I see water that a newly planted seed will use to help nourish itself and convert sunlight into energy and grow into a tree resplendent with fruit to feed the hungry." "I see the water necessary for the hydraulic system to work and to make a machine function properly." "I see water that can be used to cool the laser drill that will create new materials for high tech systems." "I see the water in a thermometer to measure the temperature of a future patient with sepsis."

As you can see by now, the possibilities are infinite. You need only to relax, open your mind, forget about stereotypical conditioned responses, and simply utilize the magnificence of your brain.

Clear your mind of thought and let the new thought surface into your consciousness (see the chapter on certainty).

A little while ago, I made an important statement. In addition, it is one of the main points of this chapter. I am referring to setting yourself above and ahead of everyone else. I stated, "You don't want to be mediocre. You want to be and need to be a standout." This might seem a little obvious and simplistic. But you must remember that the competition for entrance into medical school is not the same as the competition to get into college, unless you are applying to a top-tier 1 percent university. Now that you are applying to medical school, you are competing with the cream of the cream—thousands of medical-school applicants, and almost every one of them displays excellence. So how do you get noticed?

Reading, absorbing, assimilating, and applying the objective suggestions that I have given you throughout this book is only part of it.

Reading, absorbing, assimilating, and applying the subjective suggestions is the key to setting yourself above the rest.

These are the suggestions, tips, and pearls that will not only make you look like a better medical-school applicant but will actually mold you into a better medical-school applicant by making you into a better human being.

A medical-school applicant, a future doctor, must be compassionate; passionate; superiorly educated; dedicated; altruistic; and a focused, lifelong self-learner.

Many people go through life looking at, and seeing, only the obvious. They see only what their senses tell them. They are not skillful or creative at interpreting what they see. This is the glass-half-full versus a glass-with-liquid-in-it (and what one can do with it) perspective. That which sets certain individuals above and beyond all of the rest is their ability to not only see the set of circumstances but to be able to interpret these circumstances in view of their entire life experiences or applying knowledge that they have previously obtained in interpreting the new circumstances.

A classic example of this is at a crime scene. The victim and witnesses will report what they have seen, or think they have seen, at the time of the incident. A good policeman or detective will be able to see beyond the obvious; and, using his or her experiential skill set, he or she will be able to tell a different and much more accurate story than that which at first seemed so obvious.

Another context you can place this is in something very near and dear to you—the world of medicine.

As doctors we always have to be aware of the way we perceive and interpret information. Sometimes, that which seems obvious *is* obvious. At other times, that which seems obvious is entirely not what it seems; rather, it is a distractor to the information that we are not perceiving or interpreting correctly.

We have a saying: "Don't miss the forest for the trees." What this means is that sometimes we spend an excessive amount of time and energy concentrating on some small detail (perceptual narrowing), and we lose sight of what is around us. This is dangerous in medicine. It can happen when we focus on a single lab value's interpretation and correction while losing sight of the condition of the patient.

Another saying we have, which is the corollary of the first is, "Don't lose sight of the tree in the middle of the forest." I am sure you understand what this means, but a simple explanation would be that, although the patient has a lot going on and may have many simultaneous issues, we can't forget to look for the little things—the one little thing that may be the difference between life and death.

By now you can see how the glass-half-full/half-empty versus glass-with-liquid-in-it analysis can pertain to so many different and interesting aspects and pursuits in your life.

Just remember that first impressions are just that. Stop and assess the situation. Take a deep breath. Take a moment to slow things down. Then look at what is before you—again. What do you see? What is there in front of you that you are seeing but not interpreting correctly? What is there in front of you that you are not seeing? And lastly, what are you not seeing and need to find, see, and interpret?

This is just a handy way for you to clear the fog when you most need to. Also, this will come in handy when you are asked the tough questions (even at your interview) and don't have a lot of time to think out the answers. Trust me, you must always think with a clear head and be able to interpret the sensory input that life and medicine present to you.

It is a far better path, with far better universal consequences, to earn your position in life by your words, actions, and deeds than it is to get your position by speaking poorly, acting poorly, or even thinking poorly of others, which is another glass-half-full situation.

I have no doubt that you are familiar with the expression, "What goes around comes around."

This is a concise expression of a universal truth, and you do want your universal truths to be positive and insightful and to contribute to the well-being of your loved ones, patients, and community.

So if we believe—and up until now it has held true—that every action has a reaction, then we can say that every action is a cause, and it has a definite effect. In fact, every cause has a very definite effect.

The tough part is that the effect will not always be immediate. But trust me, everything that you say, think, and do has a consequence. Think about it. In your life, hasn't this universal truth always held up? Maybe not immediately, but somewhere along the line, hasn't there always been a consequence or effect? If you can say no to this, then I contend that you either haven't been honest with yourself or haven't looked hard enough.

So believe me when I urge you to achieve greatness through your own actions and not by putting down or hurting others. Be the best you can be and earn your position in life by your words, actions, and deeds. Success should not be determined by the failure of others.

Medicine is not about self-advancement as a result of the sacrifice of others—far from it. Medicine is about self-sacrifice for the advancement of others.

Those of you who haven't done so yet, throw away the premed mentality, which is the mentality of pushing forward no matter the consequences—the take-no-prisoners mentality. Here is a little secret: Once you get into medical school, you are no longer competing for grades. Medical school is all about learning as much as you can to be the best doctor you are capable of being. That's the secret.

This is the kind of stuff that will set you in front of all others. It is the kind of stuff that will allow you to soar above the masses, the kind of stuff that will bring you to the attention of any medical-school admissions committee.

In fact—and not amazingly—this is the type of thinking that will enable you to be very successful in life. Thinking outside of the box and considering new ways of solving problems will enable you to have a successful career and contribute to your ultimate success as a physician. In fact, it is the way civilization, as a whole, advances.

I have introduced a few interesting and significant concepts in this chapter. I started with not seeing the cup half full or half empty but rather encouraging you to see a glass with a liquid in it and allow your mind to free flow and come up with all of the possibilities. This is really just another way to encourage you to develop your skills of thinking out of the box. It is a way of encouraging you to see what is in front of you and not just accepting what you see but rather interpreting what you see and what you don't see while factoring in your vast resources of knowledge and experience. You are not just another being in the sea of mediocrity who asks "Why?" Rather, you strive for excellence by asking "Why not?"

5. You Have Nothing to Fear but Fear Itself

—FDR 1933

So, you want to be a doctor? What specialty?

Do you want to become an internist, a surgeon, or a radiologist? Perhaps you prefer to be an obstetrician or gynecologist? Have you considered a career as a gastroenterologist, pulmonologist, or a dermatologist? And then there is the long, arduous training to become a neurosurgeon, plastic surgeon, or cardiothoracic surgeon.

That's a whole lot of stuff to think about! If you are being asked this question before you've even gotten into medical school, it might be a little difficult to answer. Right now, after looking at so many options, you just might be feeling a little overwhelmed—or a lot overwhelmed. I know if anyone had asked me to pick a specialty when I was a young premed student, I probably would have completely freaked out.

So what's new? Big deal!

If you are going to get yourself accepted into medical school and become a doctor, you are pretty much going to feel overwhelmed all of the time.

That's right. Once you get into medical school, you are still going to feel overwhelmed. In fact, you are going to feel overwhelmed almost all of the time throughout your entire medical career. It doesn't even matter which specialty you choose to enter and eventually practice. Each medical specialty has its own set of stressors. So embrace it, enjoy it, and live it. Use your sense of being overwhelmed to your advantage and harness it.

Feeling overwhelmed from professional and scholastic activities is not the same as feeling overwhelmed and hopeless in life. The key is to know and understand the difference.

Feeling overwhelmed from professional and scholastic activities is a healthy expression of knowing your limitations and realizing that even with as much as you know, there is a whole heck of a lot more out there that you don't know. That is a humbling realization.
However, feeling overwhelmed and hopeless in life is an unstable and dangerous state to be in. If you feel this way now (or at any time in the future), please seek professional help and counseling. This is bad stress.

Bad stress can lead to chronic illness such as heart disease and stroke. Furthermore, if it is acutely overwhelming, it can lead to self-injury or even worse. So please, seek professional assistance and counseling if you are currently in this category.

Feelings of being professionally and scholastically overwhelmed are healthy feelings and provide you with "good" stress. This good stress is the kind of stress that gives you a jolt of the hormone cortisol and simultaneously increases levels of the hormones epinephrine and norepinephrine, the so-called fight-or-flight hormones. These are the hormones that increase your levels of readiness. They increase your physical abilities by providing heightened strength, enhanced reflexes, and diminished reaction to pain. In addition, cortisol, epinephrine, and norepinephrine will also increase your alertness and mental clarity.

Cortisol, epinephrine, and norepinephrine are really good stuff to have on board and circulating throughout your body when you need them.

The trick is to realize when you are feeling acute good stress and to use it. Good stress is an excellent resource to use to your own advantage in whatever place and situation that you want to respond to with greater clarity, certainty, productivity, and our very good friend focus (yep, focus—it just keeps showing up.).

You have known this all along; you just have not given it any conscious thought. You have put yourself in the situation to use good stress many, many times throughout all of your school years. This is the very essence behind cramming for exams, cramming for life, and being productive. In fact, it is this good stress that powers our most successful academic achievers.

This is also the very essence of athletic training. By constantly stressing our skeletons and muscles with good stress, we develop speed, agility, strength, alertness, and endurance. In addition, constant doses of good stress that come with athletic training help us to become accustomed to and prepared for the psychological stress of the actual sporting event.

We can't continuously operate at a very high level of physical and psychological stress. We are just not designed for it. It is just too much for the body and mind to handle. If you exceed your limits, you will crash and burn.

A successful way to avoid crashing and burning, or feelings of being overwhelmed by life, is to take whatever circumstance that is causing you anxiety and deconstruct it (break it down) into little pieces.

When stress comes in little packets, we can usually deal with it little by little. If we have lots of these little packets of stress, they usually don't seem insurmountable. By looking at numerous serial or parallel events, we give ourselves the ability to work much more efficiently in the long run. However, if we are constantly dealing with little bursts of stress, we can also exhaust the whole system—literally and figuratively. As long as we constantly pay attention to and deal with the issues of life on a continuous basis, we can keep stress to a minimum and convert it into good stress.

We want to harness the good stress for our needs and not fall victim to it. A simple technique that you can use as a starting point to help you through stressful periods is to break it up into smaller segments that will enable you to reach obtainable goals with each segment. And then—eureka—before you even realize it, you have gotten through it and have completed the task.

Have you ever wondered about how marathon runners operate? I mean, let's face it—to even think about running or *racing* 26.2 miles not only sounds crazy, it *is* pretty crazy. If a marathoner were to really stop and think about racing 26.2 miles, he or she would more than likely be stopped right there in his or her tracks, paralyzed with fear just thinking about the daunting journey (literally) that he or she was about to begin. Instead, marathoners see their task as a series of five-mile runs (four of them), capped off with a 10K (6.2 miles) race. It's amazing, but this really works.

This simple trick also works for mountain climbers. Take a moment and imagine yourself standing at the base of a mountain. You know that you want to climb to the top, and yet, standing there, you begin to think about all of the work and the thousands, if not millions, of steps it will take. Some mountains take a day to climb. These are the easy ones, what they call in the business "day hikes." The more serious mountains take a couple of days or weeks or even months to climb.

So here you are, standing at the foot of a mountain; and when you look up, you realize that not only can you not see the top of the mountain, you can only see a mere glimpse of the lowest of the lowest of slopes. You then get a jolt of reality and again realize that you're only at the base of the mountain.

All of a sudden, like most climbers around the world, you begin to feel overwhelmed.

I have mentioned one of my role models earlier. His name is Peter Athans. He has summited Mount Everest more times than any American ever has—seven times—and has been given the name Mr. Everest by *National Geographic* magazine. Throw in a few filming and rescue missions (as of May 2013, a total of sixteen) on top of that, and you can understand the well-deserved international recognition he has earned.

Quite a few years ago, the universe conspired to put me in the right place and at the right time. It was to be my first climbing experience, and in retrospect, it was quite a simple task. One of those day hikes. The climb was incorporated into an Outward Bound program that I was enrolled it. The theme of that particular Outward Bound week was team building. The concept is similar to the ropes and zip-line courses that are currently in vogue and utilized by many corporations, universities, and medical schools to encourage the art of team building and team dynamics among the participants. It is a very effective tool and was created by Outward Bound decades ago.

We decided to climb, in one day, one of the so-called Fourteeners of the Presidential Mountain Range, just outside of Leadville, Colorado. As we, the participants, stood at the base of the mountain, we were *all* overwhelmed.

We had all converged on that one spot to climb a mountain. It seemed like an impossible thing to do. Each of the so-called mountain climbers in our group knew that all mountains were summitable (not sure if this is even a word). We all knew that the challenges and variables when doing so might include weather conditions, food and water supply, appropriate clothing, and other stuff of a technical nature.

Yet, we were paralyzed. We just stood there. We didn't know what to do.

It was at that exact moment when the universe conspired and initiated a series of events that were to change my life—and now yours!

As the group of us stood there whining, complaining, and feeling utterly overwhelmed, we heard a strange sound. We heard someone whistling some unidentifiable tune. And then he appeared around a bend on the trail. Immediately, we all sensed that our worlds were about to change dramatically. There before us stood the epitome of the "mountaineer." To give you a visual, just think of the cover of *Outside* magazine or a Patagonia catalog. There before us, the universe had placed Peter Athans.

The funny thing was, none of us knew who he was—yet.

He stood there and just looked us over for a few minutes. It appeared that he was absorbing the moment. He then closed his eyes for a moment, and when he slowly opened them again, it felt like Yoda was looking at us and through us. Each of us had the same thought: "Why is he looking directly at me, and only me?"

He then asked me (us), "How do you climb to the top of a mountain?" I (we) replied with long-winded technical jargon. He didn't move. He just stood there, staring, and slowly began to shake his head from side to side, exactly like a frustrated professor might do after a long lecture from which the students clearly did not get the point.

After what seemed like hours, but was probably only a few seconds, he uttered these familiar and astonishingly apropos words: "You climb to the top of a mountain one step at a time."

In order to reach the top of a mountain, as long and difficult as it may seem, you get there by taking a step, one step. Then you take another step and then another—one step at a time. You link a series of individual steps and add another link and then another; and you begin to see progress. It is the linking of each of the individual steps that adds up and get you to the summit.

The overwhelming task of reaching the summit of the mountain is simply taking a step—the first step.

The secret to overcoming any overwhelming obstacle or challenge that life throws your way is simply taking a step—the first step.

It is a simple matter of putting a bunch of steps together. Taking lots of steps. Taking lots of bunches of steps all linked together. I counted a few gazillion steps on that Outward Bound day with Peter Athans on the mountain. But as it is with so many things in life, the hardest part is taking the first step. So if you are having difficulty with a task, an assignment, or making a special phone call, gather your strength, focus, and go ahead—take that first step.

What holds us back? What makes us hesitate? What stops us right in our tracks before we even take that first step to anything? What stops the majority of people? What stops *you*? Is it a lack of opportunity? Is it that you don't have the resources? Is it that other people are discouraging you? Or are you just not an optimist?

When you stop to think about it, all of these negatives have a common denominator. It is a common denominator that is not an essential part of the human condition. It is something that we are not born with but rather learn early in life, most of the time from our own life experiences. This can be a healthy adaptation to our environment, akin to the good stress that we just talked about. It can be a means for survival and self-improvement.

Unfortunately, we often don't learn this from our own experiences but rather buy into what others impose upon us. Let me get to the point. What I am talking about is fear. Yep, it is as simple as that. Fear.

Once again, we have "good fears," which we have acquired for survival, and then there are the "bad fears." These are the unreasonable, irrational fears that were usually not ours to begin with but became part of our reality. I am not a psychiatrist, and therefore I am not going to go any deeper into this subject other than to say that the way to get through these fears is to take the first step and realize that the majority of our fears are baseless. Take the first step, followed by another step, and another, and another...

Here is a little tip to dwell upon when you are faced with one of your bad fears. Reflect upon the word "fear" itself. FEAR = **F**alse **E**vidence **A**ppearing **R**eal. How profound is that? Pretty cool, simple, and true. I promise you that if you reflect upon this every time you face one of your good fears *or* bad fears, it will help you deal with the situation and make it much easier to deal with any obstacle or challenge that you face. In your daily dealings with obstacles and challengers, knowing about FEAR will help you to move forward. You won't be paralyzed, and you will be able to make wise, informed decisions. You will feel secure in your choices. You will be able to take that oh-so-critical first step.

What is the difference between a coward and a hero?

Both the coward and the hero, when exposed to danger, the great threat of bodily harm, or public speaking (the number one fear in the United States), feel fear. Cowards are stopped in their tracks. They are overwhelmed by their fears. They are reactive. They cannot move forward or accomplish the task at hand. Heroes are stopped in their tracks (momentarily). They are overwhelmed (momentarily). They readily admit their fears. They are proactive. They take the first step, and then they move forward.

Go ahead and take that first step to your medical future.

Now, getting back to my original question to you at the beginning of this chapter: Do you want to become an internist, a surgeon, or a radiologist? Perhaps you prefer to be an obstetrician/gynecologist? Have you considered a career as a gastroenterologist, pulmonologist, or a dermatologist? And then there is the long and arduous training to become a neurosurgeon, plastic surgeon, or cardiothoracic surgeon.

There is no right answer. You can choose to be whatever you choose to be. In fact, you will probably flip-flop and change your mind so many times that you won't even be able to count the changes. The good news is that it is too soon for you to come up with a reasonable medical-career choice this early in the game. The really good news is that you can always change your mind, because it is never too late. Let me repeat this last point and emphasize it because it just might save your life. Really!

You can always change your mind, because it is never too late.

Let me ask you a question. If you could wake up tomorrow morning and do whatever you wanted to do, whenever you wanted to do it, and keep doing it as much as you wished to, what would it be?

Would you choose to be a rock star? Would you want to be a professional skier? Maybe you would choose to be an internationally famous artist. Or maybe you would even decide to be the captain of a schooner plying the warm, azure waters surrounding the Polynesian archipelago. Wow, don't all of those life and career choices sound incredibly great?

I ask you, "Why not?"

Why wouldn't you drop everything and go for it? Live your dream? Some people do.

What I am trying to do is to encourage you, almost beg you, to make your career choice with the same intention. Do what you love, follow your dream, and live that dream. There is nothing better than to wake up each morning with a smile on your face. What could be better than to totally and completely love your life? Wouldn't it be total bliss if you had a job that didn't feel like a job but rather was something as enjoyable and fulfilling as the fantasy lifestyles that I mentioned above?

Think about how wonderful it would be to live each day to the fullest. How amazing it would be to live a life with passion, a life with 100 percent fulfillment.

You will live a long and happy life if it is a life of passion, joy, and fulfillment.

Unfortunately, the reality is that medical professionals have a one in three (33 percent) incidence of impairment due to drugs or alcohol.

Why is this? What is the reason? The answer is that there are a few components. First of all, and of great significance, the medical life is a life of great (and frequent) stress. The good stress helps us and should be welcomed. Unfortunately, there is an abundance of the bad stress. I have already addressed this significant issue earlier in this chapter.

The second reason is that medical professionals have access to drugs—very strong and dangerous drugs. This omnipresent access exists in spite of the abundant checks and balances that have been instituted by federal and state governments as well as federal and state medical governing bodies.

The third and foremost reason is that there are too many medical professionals who are unhappy with their careers as doctors, their chosen specialties, and their lives in general.

The medical profession has one of the highest suicide rates. This high suicide rate is right up there with air traffic controllers. So, as I have been alluding to all along, to make the choice to become a doctor is not an easy decision. To make this decision based on someone else's expectations of you, or for you, is a poor move.

To make this decision without a sense of self-sacrifice, passion, and compassion will set you up for disaster from the get-go.

Please remember, *it is never too late to change your mind.* It is never too late to change your mind and do something else. It is never too late to change your choice of specialty.

I also strongly encourage you to have hobbies. Of all of my colleagues, the ones who seem to be the happiest are those who have interests outside of the medical field. I don't mean watching television or going to the movies. I am referring to interests that take effort, such as golf, tennis, skiing, duck decoy modeling, quilting, gourmet cooking, painting, writing, and the list goes on and on. It also doesn't hurt that many of my happiest colleagues have a warm, giving family life, too.

Hobbies will give you an outlet to release or forget your stress and anxieties. Hobbies give you a means to focus on something else for a while. Hobbies give you a vacation, a reprieve, and an escape for your brain.

Trust me, you will need to escape from time to time. Even rock stars need an escape. Why do you think that we always hear about them flitting around the Caribbean Islands, which happen to be a great place to forget about the world for a while?

So, learn to escape. Who knows, maybe you can become a golf professional or an Olympic skier when you retire.

6. Role Models

We all have role models, or at least we are supposed to. Every day we read about role models in magazines and newspapers. We hear about them on the news and on the morning talk shows. Dr. Oz and Dr. Phil have built their careers around being role models. It's great that they both happen to be doctors. And the queen of role models has built a multilevel corporate conglomerate on the strength and power of being a role model. In fact, she is now one of the most famous and wealthiest women in the United States. Now that she has launched her Oprah Winfrey Network on cable TV, it will be hard to even predict what will happen next for Oprah Winfrey. Boy, does she have focus. (Focus. See what I mean? If you don't, then reread the chapter on focus.)

What is a role model? According to *Merriam-Webster's Dictionary*, a role model is "a person whose behavior in a particular role is imitated by others," or, alternatively, "someone whom another person admires and tries to imitate."

Robert K. Merton, professor of sociology at Columbia University, received the National Medal of Science for his founding of the field of the sociology of science. In his research on medical students, he stated that people want to compare and associate their behavior to a reference group that inhabits the social level to which they aspire.

In fact, I often have medical students who come by my office or send me an e-mail, asking me how to choose what specialty they should go into. This is another form of role modeling. I always tell them that when the time is right, they will know. The ivory-tower people administer medical-career aptitude tests to medical students starting in the first months of their first year. I ask myself, "Why would they want to do that so early in a medical-school education? Why would they want to perceptually narrow their thoughts, dreams, and goals so early on? Why would they want to encourage any medical student to lose his or her expansive view of medicine and medical education at such an early point?"

A medical student should focus—or, in this case, *defocus*—and try to learn as much as he or she can about everything. A medical student should be a sponge and try to absorb it all. Medical students never know what they have to know, when they have to know it, or how they will use it. A medical student's job is to learn *everything*. In fact, a premedical student's job is the same—to learn as much of everything that he or she can. (There is a lot more discussion on this in the chapter "Stop Studying for Exams.")

For most medical students, there comes a time, somewhere during the third and fourth years, when they begin to panic. They lose sleep. They lose their appetites. Rings appear under their sunken eyes. They worry and question their very existence. They ask themselves and each other, "What specialty am I going to go into?" It is during this time of high anxiety that the body's natural stress hormones, epinephrine (adrenaline) and cortisol, are released. These hormones can be destructive and a cause of many medical diseases and illnesses. But they can also be constructive and help the body adapt to the situation, or stress, at hand. The release of these hormones is part of the result of the fight-or-flight phenomenon. Epinephrine and cortisol, when utilized as positive stress, serve to heighten our senses, augment our sensory feedback, and markedly enhance our ability to interpret our surroundings.

It is during these times of benign stress that we are more receptive to environmental signals that we otherwise may not have been aware of. In the case of medical students, and all students, it is this very phenomenon that enhances learning and retention of information during "cram" studying.

It is also this heightened awareness of surroundings and increased ability to interpret that makes picking a specialty during this period of medical-school training the best time to do so. It is during this hyperaware period that medical students will see their preceptors, attendings, residents, and even their patients in a different light.

As far as preceptors, attendings, and residents are concerned, medical students will pick up on every subtle innuendo of voice and body language. They will hear inflections of the voice and slight leanings of the body that they normally never would have noticed. They will see and hear the excitement that these senior doctors demonstrate for their chosen specialties. Or—and hopefully not too often—they will bear witness to boredom, frustration, and lack of enthusiasm of their would-be role models.

Third- and fourth-year medical students will also witness the relationship that their senior doctors have with their patients. Do they see passion and compassion? Do they see a willingness and excitement to be there night and day, rain or snow, weekends or holidays? Or do they see someone who would rather be anywhere but with his or her patients?

It is this role modeling of the preceptors, attendings, and residents that is most influential and critical in the career and specialty choices of medical students.

Let me repeat: medical students pick their specialties based on role models!

And so will you! After all, aren't you basing much of your decision to become a doctor on role models whom you have had the privilege of knowing or observing?

Julius Caesar, Maimonides, Leonardo da Vinci, Thomas Aquinas, Napoleon Bonaparte, George Washington, Mahatma Gandhi, and Martin Luther King Jr. are just a few of history's role models. Through our history we have seen warriors and peacemakers. We have seen artists and scientists. Sometimes a single role model embodies all of these qualities and more.

A prime example would be Manfred, king of Sicily, 1258–1266. His was truly a benevolent and enlightened king, which welcomed all philosophies, religions, and free speech. It's a shame that we don't learn about him in American schools.

As you can see, just the few role models I have listed demonstrate how historic events may dictate who a role model may be at any given time. Throughout history, the people whom we have considered our role models have been amazingly diverse. Perhaps we might consider our role models to be evolving along with us and the particular culture that we live in.

Role models not only vary greatly over time, they also have significant cross-cultural differences. I strongly doubt that any American president of the last few decades has been a role model in the Middle East. I would also venture to guess that few Americans view Vladimir Putin, president of Russia, as a role model.

Let's not forget that one person's saint is another person's sinner. And to take that one step further, let's not forget what Oscar Wilde had to say on the subject: "Every saint has a past, and every sinner has a future." Hmm, sounds like present-day American politics.

Even as I write this, more than a few members of the House of Representatives, the US Senate, and governors are under investigation or have been sentenced to jail. There's no need to name names, because every few months, there is a whole new set of them.

We need to be careful whom we choose as role models. Our role models are sent to us; or, in the case of medical education, we are sent to them, to teach us not just the obvious medical lessons but also those not so obvious. It is their spirit, their soul, their passion, their compassion, their joy, and their heartache that shouts to us and resonates deeply within us—touching our souls.

Sometimes we are lucky enough to have the opportunity to spend a lot of time with our role models, and the lessons just rub off. This is the "do as I do" approach. We often call this the "see one, do one, teach one" approach. Words may not even be exchanged; it is just the power of the unspoken word that disseminates all of the information. At other times it may be direct lecturing from a teacher to a student. This is a concrete, defined method to transmit information and one that we are all accustomed to; however it doesn't speak to the soul.

There is also the lifetime role model. We all have one or more of these. It may be a parent, an aunt or uncle, or a grandparent. So, keep your eyes open and stay alert. You just never know when or where you are going to meet your role models. They are very rare gems, few and far between.

Let me introduce you to a few of the role models in my life and the specific lessons I have learned from them. Allow me to share with you the ingredients in the crucible that formed me and molded me to be the physician, educator, and professional advisor that I am today. Don't worry; they have already destroyed the mold. The world can only put up with one of me. These are examples to help you in seeing and recognizing your own role models—past, present, and future.

My first role model was Mr. Marion Novak. He was my sixth-grade teacher at Harbor Hill Elementary School. In those days, sixth grade didn't make the grade (pun intended) for middle school. In fact, we didn't have middle school. We had junior high school. Well, anyway, for the first few days of the school year, my classmates and I made fun of his name. After all, didn't everyone know that Marion was a girl's name? He never responded to the whispers and giggles. He never let on that he knew just what all of the passed paper notes were all about (remember that this was decades before smart phones, texting, and Twitter were even dreamed of). He just carried on in his cool and *focused* (this word is going to pop up a lot, so get used to it) way.

One day we learned about Francis Marion, the "Swamp Fox," who was one of the greatest commanders and heroes of the American Revolution. What was really amazing to my sixth-grade class was that this hero of the American Revolution, this man among men, had *two* girl's names. Imagine that—and not coincidentally, one of those two girl's names was Marion—just like our teacher, Mr. Marion Novak. From that day on, we never snickered again about the name Marion. Or perhaps it was the fact that Mr. Novak was six feet two inches tall, barrel-chested, and all of 275-plus pounds.

This fierce, gentle giant brought us to places around the world, created math wizards out of all of us, and took us on the coolest field trips. He was an expert in Renaissance literature and art. Throughout my entire life, the lessons I learned from my first role model have borne the sweetest of fruit. The most important seed that he planted into my fertile mind was to have compassion for the needs of others and passion in all of my pursuits. Hmm, are you beginning to see how important the right role models can be? Compassion and passion are two traits that are so critical for a physician to embody. These are also two extremely important traits for a future doctor applying to medical school to embody and clearly demonstrate.

Then there was Dr. Paul Calabrisi, professor of anatomy at the George Washington University School of Medicine. It was during my first week as a freshman undergraduate at GWU that I joined the premedical society. Yes, I am one of those people who always knew that I was going to be a doctor. I always had that *focus*. Anyway, the Premedical Society went on a field trip to the "old" George Washington School of Medicine located in what was then a pretty bad part of Washington, DC. The school was one hundred years old at that time, multistoried with rickety stairwells, dark corners, and...well, let me just say it was right out of a 1930s Dracula movie.

Our little group was ushered into a small, musty, dimly lit room. I noticed that there were glass bottles, containers, and tanks surrounding us. I was horrified when I came to the shocking realization that all of these glass bottles, containers, and tanks contained preserved body parts: organs and parts of organs, limbs and parts of limbs. They were all around me on stands, tables, and shelves. Just as my imagination was beginning to get the better of me—were these cut up bodies from premed students who didn't get into medical school?—there was a soft shuffle behind me and a polite cough. I jumped out of my seat and cried out. They were here for me. They were going to cut me up. I finally got ahold on myself, and I turned around to the source of the terrifying sound. There, with a ray of sunlight shining from the window, creating a heavenly conical dust mote that surrounded him in heavenly light (think Renaissance painting), was this neatly attired, diminutive man with a perfectly trimmed, pencil-thin mustache and very neatly combed, thinning gray hair. His perfectly starched, long white lab coat had his name embroidered on it: Dr. Paul Calabrisi.

For the next hour, he calmly and precisely described the steps that were necessary to get into medical school (1970s). He talked about how to develop oneself and build the perseverance necessary to become the best doctor possible. It was exactly then that I realized I had met the man who would be my mentor, my friend, and my role model. From that day on, I regularly checked in with Dr. C to maintain a steady diet of encouragement and to build my "perseverance" to enable me to achieve my long-sought-out goal. This wonderful role model helped hundreds of future doctors to see things through to the end and achieve their individual goals.

A decade later, I started my first residency. As I have said earlier in this book, you really have to want to be a doctor, and you must have...

wait for it...focus. So, ten years later, I was in my first residency in otolaryngology (they should give out awards for just being able to say the darn word). The chair of the department of otolaryngology at the University of Miami, Jackson Memorial Hospital, was James Ryan Chandler—"J. R." to those close to him and "the old man" to those not so close or to those who wanted to end their medical careers early. He was an imposing figure, known to make his residents cry—both male and female. He truly was a workaholic. He was the "Energizer Bunny" of surgery. He was indefatigable and steadfast, a perfection-ist, a magician, and a prolific writer of publications (at my last count, greater than 150). He was demanding of himself, and he expected all of these same qualities in his residents.

Working with JR was stressful, with early morning rounds at 5:00 a.m. and then a blistering day of clinics and surgeries, followed by afternoon rounds. Do you think that it was over then? Nope, guess again. Then there was admitting his patients to the hospital, get-ting them worked up, and tuning them up; and on top of all that was emergency room call. And this was all at Jackson Memorial Hospital in Miami, Florida, which was known to have the busiest emergency room in the United States. Let's just say that during this period of my life, I needed very little additional exercise, and the "Jackson Diet" was a guaranteed weight loss plan.

Getting back to J. R., he used to drill into his residents every day how important it was to be totally and completely prepared—always and without exception, no matter what. You can only imagine how that went over with us, his residents.

As you must certainly know, surgeons are characteristically OCD (which somehow sounds nicer than spelling it out). J. R.'s advice was like a narcotic for us. He fed our addiction to orderliness. He was a master. In fact, one of his favorite and often repeated sayings was, "Fifteen minutes of preparation will result in hours of surgery; hours of preparation will result in fifteen minutes of surgery." I always added, "Give or take." He was relentless in drilling this into us. Part of this process was to visualize the surgical procedure. It was our task to mentally see the surgery over and over and over again. In our minds we would create the atmosphere, the tension, the sounds, and the smell of surgery. We would walk around the hospital looking like raving lunatics as we surgically incised the air, clamping invisible blood vessels, tying sutures in the wind, and assiduously closing invisible skin.

Visualization, what a powerful tool!

Focus on the events and actions to come!

Be *certain* of your result before you even begin!

What a gift for one human being to impart to another. Don't forget, he had already drilled into us the lifelong treasure of always being exceptionally prepared down to the most miniscule of details.

Pari passu (I had to use this phrase again somewhere) to paying great attention to details, he also drummed into us that "Perfection is the enemy of good." Always make it good—very, very good. Don't be driven to perfection. Because if you are, you will destroy whatever you have created, be it surgery, art, or discussing a point of conversation. *Especially remember this, future surgeons.*

Another aspect of our surgical training with J. R. was the "commando procedure." Upon mention of this procedure, I am sure that any surgeon who is a parent or relative of yours reading this book over your shoulder, or maybe on his or her own (he or she really does care about you), just gave a sudden reflexive shudder. The dreaded commando. This is a procedure in which at least half of the patient's neck, jaw, tongue, floor of the mouth, throat, and larynx (voice box) are removed with the intention of removing cancer. This procedure is drastic and is an extreme measure to cure a very bad cancer of the head and neck—or, at the very least, to prolong the patient's life. And believe it or not, it often works. We would do a few of these each week. Sometimes back to back, ten to fifteen hours. We had to train for these, eat for these, and hydrate for these as if we were going to run a marathon. Except the marathon is easier; it only takes three and a half to four hours if you are an average runner and have trained properly. And you just don't do marathons back to back unless you are a little crazy.

What we did learn was endurance, to see things through to the very end, preparation, visualization, and, yep, here it comes again, focus. And J. R. taught us these lessons over and over. He groomed us all to become successful surgeons, leaders in our medical environments, and contributors to our communities. What a powerful role model.

Oh, and BTW, to date I have completed ten marathons and twelve half-marathons, thanks to "the old man." Oops, it slipped out.

I will now take you back to the beginning, to my first and most influential role model. He was there from the very beginning part of my life until well into my adulthood. He is an integral part of my earliest memories, stretching way back to when I was two years old. He was just always there. In fact, even today, when I face obstacles and tribulations, I ask myself what he would advise me to do. What did he teach me that I can apply to this difficult situation that I am facing? He was a major force in my life, and he was also benign and illuminating. He was a light in the darkest of times and an exemplary beacon in the best of times. This man was my grandfather Benjamin Singer (1898–1995).

He was born during an era of gas lamps and transportation by foot or horse, in a time when much of Manhattan was still a forest. He was the one who answered my childhood questions with patience and in such a way that an inquisitive idealist of a child would not lose his dreams by learning the "truth of life" too soon. We used to play chess and Scrabble together, all the while talking about current events around the world and the miracles of modern science. At times he took me on journeys into the imagination, where we explored jungles and climbed mountains together. Then we graduated to the TV show *Jeopardy*. He always waited for me to "phrase the correct response," and when I couldn't, he always had the correct response. Always. He was never wrong. He always had the correct response. It was really a shame that he wasn't alive for the popular TV game show *Who Wants to Be a Millionaire?* He would have cleaned up.

When I was in college and medical school, he was like a private consultant. He just had all of the answers. All of this from a New York City newspaper typesetter who never went to high school. Yep, there was a time when there was someone who actually had to manually arrange the individual block letters in little boxes to form the pages to be run through the printing press to create the daily newspapers. It goes without saying that this all happened long before the days of computers and immediate access to information highway of the Internet.

You might ask, "No education? How did he get so smart?" And then you might ask, "Where can I buy some of this secret stuff?" Well, the answer, my friend, is right in front of you and always has been. He read and read, and then he read some more. In fact, he read everything that he ever helped print and as much of everything else that he could get his hands on.

This wonderful man, this role model, taught the lesson that through consistent study and the steady accumulation of knowledge over many years, one acquires the backbone and the crucible for discovery, self-growth, and lifelong learning. His legacy as a role model was to instill the ability and knowledge to answer the questions and solve the problems that the greatest journey of all—life—may put on your path as you travel toward your dreams and goals.

So as you can see, role models can be—are—extremely important in the process of developing into who we will eventually become. If you make poor choices in your role models or choose them for the wrong reasons—the quick fix, dirty money, instant gratification, or to be "cool"—you can be led down a road of self-destruction. Choose them right, and you can be molded and prepared for a life of fulfillment and happiness.

I already suspect that you have been careful in your choice of role models, for really, who has influenced you and guided you here to this point in your education? Who has inspired you? Who has created your "inner doctor"? I would like you to stop reading for a moment. Close your eyes and just let the images of your role models appear in your mind. See them, feel them, smile with them, and then thank them.

Once you have established your role model—or hopefully role models, as in many—then what? This isn't something that you have to ask about. It comes automatically. Your role models become, in Freudian parlance, your superego. The superego seeks perfection. It keeps you on the straight and narrow. It is your inner voice that keeps you from giving into narcissistic satisfaction. Referring back to a popular motto of the 1990s, WWJD ("What Would Jesus Do")?

At this point you are probably asking yourself, "What the heck is this guy talking about, and what does this have to do with me getting into medical school?"

The first lesson that any role model should have taught us is to do the right thing. We are faced with a constant barrage of obstacles and challenges, and therefore decisions, throughout the day, every day. When your response is automatic, and feels right, it *is* right (unless you are a sociopath, but that is a subject for another place and another time). When you hesitate with your response, when something just doesn't feel right, it *isn't* right. This should be ingrained into the very depths of your soul. This is a significant part of the human condition. Trust it! Always!

So, getting back to our role models, it is our role models who, by example, have demonstrated these very qualities that we wish to emulate. We want to be like them. It is the past actions of our role models that we have observed that have greatly affected all that we do and think. It is these observations and lessons that drive us forward in doing the right thing with passion, compassion, perseverance, endurance, visualization, focus, certainty, and love. I am not going to get into the last one; just go with it. It is just a little too personal. Sorry.

7. Stop Studying for Exams!

Stop studying for exams! Yes, you read that right. If ever we were to meet and you were to hear me lecture, you wouldn't have to clean your ears or go for an ear checkup. You would have clearly heard me say it, and I would have left no doubt in your mind. Maybe you would turn to the person sitting next to you and ask them, "Did he just say 'Stop studying for exams'?" Your neighbor would confirm that you did hear me correctly.

Every year I freak out the entering class of first-year medical students when I begin my very first lecture of the year with "Stop studying for exams." I say it earnestly, and eventually they begin to realize that I am 100 percent serious.

So please take my admonition to heart. Stop studying for exams! What? Am I crazy? A doctor, a medical-school educator, telling you, a student and medical-school applicant, to stop studying for exams?

What am I talking about? Aren't college and medical school all about grades? Isn't your success as a student measured by the grades that you get? Isn't your grade point average (GPA) one of the strongest measuring parameters in deeming your suitability for medical-school admission? Isn't your GPA based on your quiz grades, exam grades, and resultant course grades? Then why the heck am I extolling to you the virtue of no longer studying for your exams? Why am I saying this to you, and why have I told this to a multitude of students before you?

Because I do want you to *stop studying for exams*!

If you decided to read this book first as a medical-school applicant, and you are now rereading this chapter because I advised you to do so after being accepted to medical school, I will start with an explanation to you first.

If you are in college and are premed, I want you to read this chapter as if you were already in medical school. This is a form of method acting (making believe you are already in medical school and reacting with your actions, thoughts, and conclusions as a medical student would). So make your way through this chapter as a newly accepted applicant to medical school, and then reread this chapter after you *are* accepted to medical school. I guarantee you that each reading will be as if you were seeing these words for the very first time.

I would like you to reread this chapter every time you begin to freak out about studying for exams throughout the remainder of your time in college and medical school.

So let me say it again: *stop studying for exams*!

When you are accepted into medical school, you are being given the most wonderful *and* the most fearful gift that can be given to a human being. Better yet, you have earned the most wonderful, and the most fearful, responsibility imaginable. You will be entering into a lifetime of unconditional service. When you accept the responsibility of giving unconditional service, you take an oath to give of yourself in such a way that will require your giving unlimitable (that must be a new word) passion, compassion, love, time, sweat, and tears.

So what about the gift? What have you earned?

You have been given the gift of saving a life. You have been given the gift of saving two lives, ten lives, countless lives. On any given day, you may save a life with basic CPR. At other times you may perform skillful, unprecedented surgery. Perhaps one day you will order an antibiotic that will stop death in its tracks. Or perhaps you might pull a foreign body out of a child's throat and hear the magnificent rush of fresh air as tortured lungs refill. You might have to change a blood pressure medication from one that was marginally working to another one that gets the job done and prevents an imminent stroke.

Right about now, some of you are beginning to get an inkling of what this precious gift is and why I want you to stop studying for exams.

At times you will see the immediate effect of your actions. It will be an immediate cause to an immediate effect. At other times you will never know the effect of the action that you are causing. Sometimes there is a very apparent relationship between cause and short-term effect. Unfortunately, there are scenarios where your action does not have any effect that is visual or apparent to any of your senses.

But rest assured, every cause has an effect! It is a basic law of nature. It is one of the backbones of quantum mechanics. It is deeply rooted in metaphysical theology. It is there for all of us to see as a tenet of all the world's major religions. It is also the basis of the development of our Freudian ego. You just might not be witness to the effect. If a butterfly flaps its wings in California, might it not cause a monsoon in Asia?

But, my dear reader, right now, right now at this very moment, you are being given the gift. You are earning the gift.

The paradox is, you just never know what you have to know to be able to fulfill this magnificent destiny. In other words, you just don't know what you have to know, when you have to know it, under what circumstances you will be called upon to use it, and how much of it you will have to know.

So *stop studying for exams*! Do you get it yet?

Let's think about this a little more. If you don't study for your exams, aren't you going to be in danger of getting poor grades in school? Or perhaps you will suffer a worse fate. If you don't study for your exams, won't you be in danger of flunking? Won't your GPA go down? And then won't it be practically guaranteed that you will destroy your chances of getting into medical school?

The answer is a definitive *no*! In fact, I suspect that your grades just might improve. How can that be? How does not studying for exams improve your grades?

I keep telling you to stop studying for exams. Well, yes, I have asked you to stop studying for exams. But I haven't made myself quite clear yet, have I? So that is what I am going to do right now. I am going to make myself clear. Are you ready?

I want you, as of this moment, to stop studying for exams and to start studying for your patients.

Study for your patients!

That's it. That's all there is to it. Study for your patients. Wow! What a concept. Stop and think about it. When you finally do think about it and realize that every morsel, every tidbit, every pearl that you learn might be the one thing that you will need to remember, the one little thing that you will have to recall to save the life of that one future patient, ten future patients, one thousand future patients (and, of course, infinite generations of their progeny), you will be astounded by how much easier it will be to learn and retain information. You will be blown away by how powerful an incentive it is to learn for learning's sake. Learn for the sake of all of your future patients, their families, and their progeny for the many generations yet to come.

You just never know what you are going to need to know until you find yourself in a position that requires you to know it.

Read that last sentence a few times, and you will get it. It is a profound statement and one of the most important concepts of this entire book. That is why I keep repeating it so many times. In fact, past studies have indicated that when presented with a bit of new information—not overwhelming, sensory-taxing information—most people will retain 50 percent after the first presentation. After seeing the information a second time, most people retain 75 percent of the new information. And with a third presentation, most people will retain up to 95 percent.

This is one of the reasons why, in many hospitals and independent surgicenters, the informed consent form (the document that reviews the nature of the surgical procedure, the possible poor outcomes, and possible risks and complications) is presented three times and by three different people before the patient has the opportunity to sign his or her name to the document. This is why I keep repeating myself so much. It really works.

If you are not yet in medical school when you read this chapter, just keep reading and absorb what I am saying here. And like I said earlier, after you are accepted to medical school, come back and read it again. You will get a totally different meaning from it. And then, as I said earlier, each time you begin to freak out about an upcoming exam, come back and read this chapter again.

In fact, right after I wrote the above paragraphs, my then-twelve-year-old son asked me what I had written. I saw it as an awesome opportunity to impart my wisdom to him. I looked at him and said, "Stop studying for exams."

My then-ten-year-old daughter immediately said, "What? Are you crazy? Then why do I have to go to school?"

My son then calmly turned to her and very pedagogically (that means like a teacher) said, "What Dad means is that you shouldn't study for exams, but study to be prepared for any and all situations that come up in life." Wow. And that was from my twelve-year-old son. What an amazing moment for this proud dad. He totally got it. He got it to the point that he was able to explain it and pass it on to his ten-year-old sister. In the field of education, they say that to demonstrate that you truly understand something, you should be able to teach it to another. Anyway, she just thought we were both crazy and said that she intended to keep studying for her exams. Well, at least for now.

Another way to look at this is to realize that life is about real situations involving real people. Every day you read, see, or hear about the ecstasy and the agony of real life. In this technology-laden, overbearing communications era, we become aware of events on the other side of the continent, around the world, or in outer space almost instantly. We all have the potential to be suddenly thrown into the middle of it—the good *and* the bad.

As a doctor, you will always find yourself in a position of leadership, responsibility, and caring for the needs of others. You will be given the gift of knowledge. You will obtain the knowledge to ease the pain and suffering of others. You will have the opportunity to affect the quality of life of friends and strangers. Ultimately, it will be your destiny to save a life, ten lives, one thousand lives.

As I said earlier (and keep repeating), there is a concept so important that it is worth repeating yet again: You just don't know what you have to know, when you have to know it, under what circumstances you will be called upon to use it, and how much of it you will have to know. But the greater your knowledge base and the development of your skill sets, the better prepared you will be. It might very well be that the information presented to you in a lecture today will be a fundamental part of your core being tomorrow—even though it might seem like minutiae or trivia right now. You just don't know that today.

An example of this principle is related to a horrible and most unfortunate skin disease that is called Kaposi's sarcoma. Up until the early 1990s, when thousands of currently practicing doctors were still in medical school or residency, Kaposi's sarcoma was a mere footnote in *Robbin's Textbook of Pathology*. Mind you, *Robbin's Textbook of Pathology* was then, and still is now, one of those textbooks that is so cumbersome and heavy that you have to work out regularly to develop the strength just to carry it. This book is huge—thousands of pages long. Since the late 1980s and 1990s, thousands of pages have been written just about Kaposi's sarcoma in scientific and professional journals, as well as medical textbooks. Little did I—or any other medical student, intern, or resident back in those days—know or have even the slightest inkling that the Kaposi's sarcoma was to become a major part of the diagnosis of a current catastrophic disease that kills millions of people around the world every year and has been doing so for almost three decades. Who would have known that it was to become one of the hallmarks in the progression of HIV/AIDS? It was just a small footnote, hardly worth a few meager sentences, buried deep within the bowels of *Robbin's Textbook of Pathology*.

Another, and more personal, example occurred when I was a second-year medical student. My classmates and I had just attended a lecture on cardiac auscultation (that's listening to the heart sounds with a stethoscope; medical terminology is designed to confuse everyone else), and, mixed in with the usual run-of-the-mill heart sounds, our professor had taught us about some really unusual heart sounds. Usually, as humans, we tend to not pay attention to the minutiae and easily forget the truly rare stuff that is buried within school lessons and in life. For some reason, my professor's teachings that day on the rare stuff (what we in medicine call "red herrings") stayed with me, buried somewhere in my brain.

Six months later, while I was on winter break, I found myself practicing my ancient skills of cardiac auscultation (you know what that means now) on my family. I practiced on everyone, including my sisters, parents, and uncles and aunts. Everyone I checked sounded normal. Frankly, I was beginning to get a little bored. Then it was time for me to listen to my eighty-five-year-old grandmother's aged heart—a heart that had steadily beat billions of times over so many years. I slowly placed the diaphragm (the wide flat part of the stethoscope) on her wrinkled chest. I had difficulty hearing the distant beat. And then, almost imperceptibly, I heard something different. I didn't hear the usual lub-dub, lub-dub, lub-dub that is associated with a normal, healthy heart. My ears perked up, and my senses were primed. My focus narrowed. I strained to hear better.

Actually, our hearing literally does improve when we strain to hear better. This is very much like our vision when we need to see better. When we squint our eyes to increase our visual acuity (sharpness), we distort the lens of the eye to improve the refraction and produce a clearer image on the retina. And so with hearing, when we strain, we increase the tension on the stapedius muscle (the smallest muscle in the human body) and tighten the tensor tympani muscle (the second smallest muscle in the human body). These two muscles are anatomically located within the middle ear. With the tensing of these muscles, there is an improvement in hearing by increasing the efficiency of the eardrum and tiny middle ear bones, the malleus, the incus, and the stapes.

So there I was, straining away, trying to hear the familiar lub-dub, lub-dub, lub-dub of my grandmother's heart, but instead I heard lub-dub-dub, lub-dub-dub, lub-dub-dub. There was a third heart sound. I was alarmed and immediately asked myself, "What the heck is going on here? What is this extra sound? What is this strange, mysterious, and abnormal sound coming from my grandmother's heart?"

And then it hit me! It was like a bolt of lightning. In one of the introductory lessons about the physical examination of patients, the instructor had casually mentioned a physical finding that would be handy to know. He said that, being beginning first-year students, we need not worry about it for the time being. He even went so far as to say that this little golden nugget of knowledge wouldn't even be on any of our upcoming exams. It was at that very moment that most of my classmates completely tuned out what he was about to tell us. After all, it wasn't even going to be on any forthcoming exams. To me, his words were a beacon. It was as if a spotlight was shining on him, and he was speaking directly to me. This wasn't going to be on an exam anytime soon, but it might be helpful in the future. Hmm, there really wasn't any big decision here. I would learn for learning's sake and for the sake of my future patients.

Returning to my grandmother, here it was, that little golden nugget that I had heard in class—and it wasn't some time way out there in the future. I really surprised myself when I realized that I not only recognized this third heart sound right then and there, but I also was able to use the golden nugget in a practical way. I then proceeded to scare the "stuff" out of my grandmother and my family when I gently—nope, very excitedly—explained to her that she had a problem with her heart that she needed to take care of right away. And do you know what? She actually listened to my advice. Of course she would listen to her grandson, the doctor. The very next day, she went to see her doctor, who informed her that she was in heart failure and placed her on the appropriate medications. She went on to live a few happy years longer.

It was then that I *stopped studying for exams.*

I just didn't know what I would have to know, when I would have to know it, under what circumstances I would be called upon to use it, and how much of it I would have to know. Diagnosing my grandmother was the perfect lesson to emphasize this incredibly important concept. Thank God that everything worked out the way it did.

So much of how you react, and the appropriateness and the correctness of your actions, is based upon your experiences and knowledge. Medical education (graduate education) and the residency programs (postgraduate education) are designed to build your experiences and knowledge. As this is a book about getting into medical school, I will not describe or review residency programs.

Medical school is where you begin to build the foundation and learn the skills to become a lifelong learner. It is in medical school where you will be inundated with lecture materials, clinical skills teaching, and hands-on patient contact. All of this comes with a constant anxiety over how to manage your time to fit it all in.

Let me remind you, you are no longer going to compete to get into medical school. You are no longer going to obsessively attempt to get the highest grades possible. You are no longer going to study for exams. You are now going to do all of the above to become the best doctor that you can possibly be. You have been given the greatest gift, and you must receive it with the understanding of the responsibility that you are accepting.

So with your permission, please let me say it one more time: *stop studying for exams!*

8. Compassion and Volunteerism

One of the main characteristics sought out in medical-school applicants, our future doctors, is compassion. So many interviewers look for this as a key attribute that the medical-school applicant must have. I am referring to true compassion—compassion that is deep in their souls, burned into their very existence, and part of their very being. Walking the walk, not just talking the talk. You know, the good old-fashioned garden variety "actions speak louder than words."

You might ask how an admissions committee or an interviewer can sense such a subjective quality in the applicant. How do they evaluate this? What are they thinking? How are they going to ask applicants questions that will not, either knowingly or unwittingly, set up the applicant to give memorized, stock answers that they may have learned on the Student Doctor Network website (studentdoctor.net)?

Then you might think, *What should I be thinking? How can I show myself as the compassionate person that I really am without making my answers too melodramatic? How can I demonstrate my compassion without seeming like I am overselling myself?*

How can you identify compassion? And if identified, how can you assess and quantify compassion? There is no compassiometer, is there? Wow, if there was, we would all want to own one for when we pick our own doctors or teachers or people at the return line counter at Walmart or Chanel or Louis Vuitton. Heck, why not use a compassiometer when dating or to exchange our parents or...? Freud would have a field day with that one.

The secret is found within the contents of the application. It is revealed in the narratives, in the extracurricular activities, and even in the summer activities. The secret is really not such a big secret at all—it is really right out there in the open. Admissions committees look for a specific activity, which is an activity that we all should be involved in as human beings.

This activity should be part of our very essence of being a part of a community and society. It is what makes us part of a successful community. The secret ingredient looked for by all admissions committees as a barometer of compassion is *volunteerism*.

Volunteerism is a code word for compassion. Not as complex as the "Da Vinci code," but as in Dan Brown's novels, it is a code that is right out there in front of your nose. What exactly is volunteerism? A simple answer would be *volunteering to help others out*. But it really goes beyond this simple definition. The qualities that an admissions committee is looking for in a medical-school applicant are often demonstrated in the act of volunteerism.

Perhaps a better definition of volunteerism might be that it is an expression of willingness to undertake and commit to helping others and to do for others or a particular cause, without the expectation of receiving payment or anything else in return.

Volunteerism is giving of ourselves, utilizing our talents, our education, and our abilities, which we have received to help others and to share with others. Receiving for the sake of sharing is all about compassion.

What is medical education? It is traditionally a process, over four years, whereby a medical student learns the art and science of medicine from clinicians and researchers who share their knowledge and experience. This knowledge and experience just happen to be in the field of medicine.

During the first two years of medical school, prior to the clinical third and fourth years, students are presented with the classic subjects of anatomy, physiology, histology, microbiology, pathology, and cellular and molecular biology. In some medical schools, these subjects are taught in formal didactic lectures. In other medical schools, these subjects are taught in small-group fashion and are incorporated into a series of clinical vignettes.

Today's medical students, as part of their normal coursework, are also exposed to medical ethics and professionalism—subjects that have been ignored for decades in medical education—as part of their formal education. Medical ethics and professionalism are a critical part of medical education and the practice of medicine. In the past there was a totally inappropriate absence in medical education of such important disciplines. Doctors were basically in a free-for-all state of doing the right thing, or not doing the right thing, when it came to ethics and professionalism. This is one of the major reasons so many doctors got themselves—and, unfortunately, sometimes their patients—into trouble in the past.

As history has shown us time and time again, in the midst of darkness, there is still some light. Ethicists, religious leaders, politicians (hmm, I see the makings of an oxymoron here), teachers, and law enforcement professionals gathered and shared information to improve and add to ethics and professionalism in medical education in all medical schools across the country.

Today, medical students are educated with and receive the cumulative knowledge of countless generations of medical adepts and are entrusted with sharing this knowledge and this gift in the ministering to the needs of their community and patients.

Now let's get back to the topic of volunteerism. Do you remember the question that everyone has asked you throughout your life? You know, the one you are so sick and tired of being asked. The one that looms right there in front of you that you are going to have to answer truthfully, eventually. And if you have escaped it so far, they are going to get you with it at your interview (see chapter 18). Well, here it is, just in case you forgot. Yeah right!

Why do you want to be a doctor?

And the answer is...drum roll please...wait for it... "Because I want to help people." As I said earlier in this book, this is a lame answer. You can help yourself and others, saving time, aggravation, and stress, by becoming a plumber. Plumbers make lots of money, and they "help people" in some of their moments of greatest need (please see my earlier discussion on the economics of being a plumber).

So, do you want to help people by using a skill that is unique to a relatively small and gifted group of people? This noble professional group of people includes such illustrious names as Avicenna, Galen, Maimonides, Albucasis, Osler, Cushing, and Bernard. You see, it goes beyond helping others. It goes way beyond that. It is a mind-set, a way of living, and a way of viewing the world. What all of these great physicians had in common, and what great physicians of today have in common, is compassion.

Compassion. If you have it, it is part of you, a gift. It is the very thing that makes you do what you do, your driving force. You wake up with it, and it is with you when you go to sleep. It is the force that allows you to never question giving up those parts of your life that other people are just not willing to give up. Miss a party, leave a movie before it is over, or cancel an engagement (not the marrying kind; you are allowed to schedule around that), no problem. It is what gives you no choice when you are at Disney World with your kids and you see a commotion at the LEGO store, and you rush through the crowd to render aid and assistance to stabilize a woman having a grand mal seizure until the paramedics get there.

In a word, it is compassion. Compassion for our fellow human beings at all times, at any place, under all circumstances, without exception. This is compassion.

When you are applying to medical school, one of the key qualities that you are scrutinized for is whether or not you truly have compassion. You are not only scrutinized as to whether or not you have it, but also as to what degree you might possess it.

How do you clearly demonstrate compassion, especially if you don't want to brag or let your ego get in the way? In your essays or narratives, you don't want to go overboard, because if you push this one too hard, even if your intentions are noble, you will lose. You will undermine and negate the richly deserved impression that you have created for yourself with all of the wonderful compassionate endeavors you have been involved in or are currently actively involved in.

How do you let it be known that you are compassionate? How do you sincerely and humbly transmit this valuable attribute that you possess?

Do you remember that a little earlier, we talked about the "code," as in the Da Vinci code? Of course you do. Just in case you need a gentle reminder, the code word for compassion is volunteerism. Let's talk about this a little.

In the chapter on leadership we will talk about Habitat for Humanity and how this would be a wonderful avenue to demonstrate leadership. An effective leader leads from the front lines; an effective leader leads by example; an effective leader will get his or her hands dirty, start at the bottom, learn the ropes, help others, and work his or her way up until he or she can grow into a leadership role. A sideline of this is that, through all of the hard work, time, and sincerity that you contribute, you will also be making a difference in the world. Maybe it is a small difference overall, but it is a tremendous difference in a single family's life.

This kind of sounds like, "That's one small step for man, one giant leap for mankind" (Neil Armstrong, 1969). Wow, it doesn't get much better than that.

Actually, being a part of a project like Habitat puts a roof over a family's head, puts walls around them, supplies a kitchen in which they will be able to cook and eat, and offers a hearth around which to gather. That is compassion. What about those who are less fortunate in life? How might you help them?

There are soup kitchens in most communities. They are usually sponsored by local religious groups and civic organizations. You don't have to be a member of any particular religious institution, and for that matter, you don't have to share their religious or spiritual beliefs. What does matter is that you consistently give of yourself, feeding (literally or figuratively) those who are less fortunate and doing so on a long-term, consistent basis.

The best—and hardest—part is to seek nothing or ask for anything in return! You do it just to *do* it.

That, my friend, is the basis of volunteerism: giving without any expectation of return. Just to help others.

Another avenue for expressing your compassion is to become arms-deep in the care of the terminally ill. The institution of hospice lends itself beautifully well to the symbiotic relationship of those who are in need of much loving care and the caregiver—you—who wants to lovingly give and share.

Hospice is usually the final step in the long series of life events for the terminally ill. For many it is a respite at the end of a long, hard journey. It is a place to be surrounded by loved ones and friends. It is a place that is equipped to handle the demands and to take care of the ever-increasing daily living needs of the terminally ill.

Hospice is also adept at providing the medications that might be too difficult or dangerous for loved ones to administer. As health declines, other needs arise, such as personal hygiene, cleanliness, and nutrition. As you can see, there are plenty of opportunities for an eager, compassionate person—you—to help someone else during their time of greatest need.

This is an opportunity for you to be there, right there on the front lines of volunteerism in a one-on-one relationship with someone, an individual who needs you. I am talking about another human being who needs you more than anyone has ever needed you before.

This is a time for you to establish a relationship with someone who cannot do things on his or her own. This is a time for you to give and share of yourself in a way that you can never have imagined possible. This is a way for you to open the door, your door, of selfless giving. This is a time for you to initiate selfless giving for the rest of your life. This is an opportunity for you to demonstrate to yourself that you do have it in you to give without any expectation of receiving for yourself.

This is compassion in its purest form.

This is being a doctor.

Go ahead. Give it a try. You just might discover that it is very infectious and that you won't be able to stop.

Hmm, does this sound like a quality that we want to see in every medical-school applicant? Is this a quality that every medical-school admissions committee wants to see in every medical-school applicant? For that matter, is this a quality that all patients want to see in every doctor, and particularly in *their* doctors?

There is another very personal, special avenue for you to express your compassion. This is a unique way for you to make a huge impact and improve the quality of life for your fellow human beings who have a great need for you. Yes, that's right. They are waiting for you and your help. They are waiting right now, even as you are reading this line. What I am referring to is a population living in every community—in your town and in every town in the United States. I am referring to our fellow community members who are housebound secondary to any one of numerous circumstances, including age, somatic illness, mental illness, lack of transportation, or just great difficulty with "the system."

As you can see, this is an incredible opportunity for you to be involved, truly involved, in a one-on-one relationship with someone in need, truly in need of you. If you already are a highly compassionate person, then you already know the many ways in which you can help.

If you are just entering the world of volunteerism, scratching the surface, if you will, then you will be amazed by the joy, appreciation, and gratitude that you will receive and give. So once you find that special person who needs you (through the various social service organizations in your community), you might then ask, "What can I do?"

The good news—no, the great news—is that there are numerous opportunities out there just waiting for you.

Take, for example, the elderly, nonambulating widow(er) who is housebound, has no family, and has survived all of his or her friends. He or she will be in need of transportation to medical care visits. He or she will need someone (you) to pick up groceries and prescriptions.

Speaking of transportation to medical visits, there almost certainly will be a need for someone to coordinate medical care, including visits to his or her primary care physician and referred medical/surgical specialists. This is a golden opportunity for volunteerism.

In our aging patient population, there is an expanding need for evaluation by multiple medical/surgical specialists. As they age and enter their advanced senior years, more and more people will, more than likely, need someone to cook for them and oversee their nutritional needs. Perhaps they will need assistance in personal care and hygiene.

Unfortunately, with advancing age, there is too often an associated decline in one's ability to take care of one's personal health and hygiene, not just from a physical point of view but also from a declining mental status with loss of personal oversight. As you can see, this is a wonderful opportunity to enter into a long-term, consistent, and exceptionally beneficial act of volunteerism.

"Personal" volunteerism doesn't have to be limited to the aging population; it is also beneficial to people with chronic illnesses and some acute illnesses (e.g., after major trauma, postsurgery), the medically indigent, and those with mental and emotional issues.

Helping manage the affairs of people in their time of greatest need has another hidden opportunity for you. Think about it for a moment. Managing someone else's medical, therapeutic, hygienic, nutritional, and transportation needs is a great way to develop and demonstrate your nascent leadership skills. Wow, two for the price of one! (Please see the next chapter, "Leadership.")

So go for it. Get out there and lend a helping hand—or foot (sorry, I couldn't resist). Volunteerism is where you get to live your compassion. Volunteerism is how you will demonstrate your compassion. Volunteerism *is* compassion!

In your application and at your interview, one of the major aspects of volunteerism (compassion) that will be evaluated is your level of commitment. The medical-school admissions committee and your interviewer will evaluate the depth of your volunteer experience. Handing out magazines to patients at a hospital does not carry the same weight as medical missionary work overseas. In addition, the number of hours per week, duration of activity (weeks or months), and the responsibility of your position will be evaluated. Commitment is very important.

9. Leadership

What makes a leader, a leader?

Is a leader just someone who is in charge? Is a leader someone who simply has followers? Do we consider someone a leader if he or she is a trendsetter or stylista? Is a leader supposed to evoke feelings of fear and dread? Is a leader someone who forces others to follow with threats and intimidation?

Perhaps a leader is someone who received the most votes during an election because he or she made so many false promises and inspired a multitude of empty dreams for the voters. Hmm, sounds very familiar. Maybe the official with the most money and the best lobbying firm in tow automatically becomes the leader. That sounds even more familiar—and too close to home.

Is the team captain always the strongest, the smartest, the toughest, or, for that matter, the best athlete on the team? Is the chief always the strongest, the smartest, the toughest, or, for that matter, the best warrior in the tribe?

There is also the perennial drone who just trudges along and tediously works his or her way up the ladder to the top rung, deserved or not but put there by the rules. Hmm, that one sounds like our congressional leadership.

Can you think of any other leadership roles or leadership types that you know personally? Have you ever asked yourself how they got there? Think about it. Really. What do you think are the main reasons for how and/or why they got there?

I just thought of a really good one. This one is popular and, unfortunately, quite prevalent among medical-school applicants. Most medical-school committee members and application reviewers see it for what it really is. These are the real "gunners" among medical-school applicants who initiate or create an entirely new campus organization, club, or society just so they can become its leader. The organization's creation was constructed solely for their purposes or personal gain. It is a creation to fill in a spot on the medical-school application and to show that they have served in a leadership role and have run an organization.

This creation of a university club or organization is one of my favorites. It is one of my favorites in a less-than-positive sense—please understand that I am being sarcastic and that it is one of my least favorite things on a medical-school application. It stands out like a sore thumb. It is a red flag. It opens up a whole avenue for medical-school interviewers to explore and dissect. Believe me, the medical-school admissions committee is expert at seeing things for what they really are. With each medical school receiving a few thousand applications for the few coveted seats that they offer, they become very, very good at what they do.

Having said that, medical-school admissions committees, and interviewers in particular, are also quite expert at also discerning when a medical-school applicant has initiated or created an entirely new campus organization, club, or society for the right reasons. This type of applicant sees a need, or void, and creates out of compassion, service, or excellence.

So take a moment. Sit back. Close your eyes. Breathe deeply and relax.

What qualities do you think a leader should have? Actually, a better question would be, what qualities do you think an excellent, effective leader should have? Immediately, a whole string of questions about great leaders come to mind.

What forces come together to create a leader? What is it that galvanizes mere mortals to take charge when the going gets tough? Why do people continue to lead in the face of uncertainty? How is it that true leaders seem to be the ones who will face death when it most counts? Why is it that a great leader will manage to find time to learn about, work with, and strengthen the weakest link in any chain of people for which they are responsible, even in the midst of crises or circumstances with extreme consequences?

Have you given it a little thought? Let's see what you have come up with. What makes a leader? Or, as I asked you a minute or two ago, "What qualities do you think an excellent and effective leader should have?"

Now would be a good time for you to once again sit back, close your eyes, and come up with some answers to this question. Imagine great leaders and see them in your mind's eye. Think about the qualities that you feel have made them great leaders. Ruminate over how they became who they are/were and how some of them have been recognized nationally and internationally. What is it that has allowed still others to be recorded in the chronicles of history and be remembered for all time and by countless generations?

Now, take a few minutes and write down the names of the leaders you recognize. Some will be famous and others not so famous—a teacher, coach, or a friend, for example. List under each name the attributes and qualities that you feel make that person a great leader. When you complete this exercise, you will more than likely see a pattern—or a few patterns. After all, not all great leaders lead in the same style. And not every situation or amalgamation of circumstance calls for the same type of leadership skills.

The captain of a sailing ship will use an entirely different set of skills to command than a chief executive officer (CEO) who is running a conference. Yet they do share a few attributes in common.

It is said that a great leader leads by example. Let's explore this for a moment. Leading by example is not necessarily as altruistic as it sounds. Really, what do most parents do if not lead by example every single day? Of course, that doesn't necessarily make them great leaders.

Great leaders will not ask others to perform actions, face dangers, or risk their lives unless they themselves have demonstrated that they are willing to do the very same thing. Great leaders have a history of getting into the muddied trenches with their soldiers. Great leaders demonstrate an understanding of the needs and desires of those whom they lead.

We have all heard stories about one of the greatest leaders of American history. It is reported that George Washington used to walk among his troops on the eve of battle, exchanging words with as many of them as he could. A compliment here, a suggestion there would go a long way. He made it his mission to know little factoids about each of them. His adjutant administrative executive officer would do the research for him in advance. But to the common foot soldier, knowing that or not knowing it was of no importance or significance. The fact that the general cared to know the little details, cared to make it personal, was what solidified George Washington's whole mystique.

Then, as today, wise leaders personalize their leadership. This inspires those under them to believe in their leaders and to follow them in what seems like a personal relationship. General George Washington understood that all of the soldiers under his command had unique qualities and skills that he could enlist to achieve ultimate success in their common goal. He learned to utilize each individual by understanding his unique and individual skills.

Mahatma Gandhi is often considered one of the greatest leaders in world history. When he asked others to fast, he fasted. When he asked others to protest, he protested. What he asked of others, he did. He might have even said, "I ask of others only what I would do myself." Now, that was a nice paraphrasing of the Golden Rule.

He inspired millions to follow him and to join together as one to help solve many of the problems of the long-standing social-cultural system in India. He had a unique style of leadership. He had an uncanny skill of successfully encouraging his millions of followers to believe in themselves and their dreams. He preached that in pursuing their dreams, they could collectively accomplish the impossible and that it was the right thing, and the just thing, and the righteous thing to do. The masses, the millions, did not hesitate to follow him. He taught people to believe and, through belief, to collectively achieve.

On any given weekend during football season, a group of forty-three players is activated for the game, and a group of eleven players takes the field at any time. These are big guys—big in stature and big in ego. If they were leaderless, they would be like a ship without a rudder, and more than likely they would flounder on the sea of green grass or artificial turf.

Keep in mind that each player is a specialist and a standout in his own right. Each one of the big guys was chosen to be on the team to perform a specific task. All of the big guys are specialists, and their specialties are needed to accomplish what is required for the team to move the ball forward a few yards and put points on the scoreboard. How are they kept in line and brought together as a collective group to accomplish such a Herculean feat?

Take Tom Brady, Peyton Manning, or any of the great quarterbacks of the NFL, past, present, and future. Why are they leaders akin to generals on the battlefield? What leadership skills do they exemplify? NFL quarterbacks clearly demonstrate the concept of leadership by example. Throughout every game and practice, week after week, they call the shots—and they take the big shots. They also have to be decisive, be quick-thinking, have a positive attitude, and read the ever-changing circumstances that they face on the field at any given moment. The quarterback must be able to organize and bring together really big guys. But above all that, the quarterback is there, right in the middle of the melee, taking his hits. The great quarterbacks lead by example.

Being able to demonstrate your leadership skills without blowing your own horn is an important quality to nurture. There are many life circumstances, either elective or nonelective, in which you will be called upon to do so. Of course, on your medical-school application, there is plenty of opportunity for you do so. In fact, on the medical-school application, they ask you very directly to list your past leadership roles. This is in the section where you list your past life experiences. Many secondary medical-school applications ask you, once again, to list your past leadership experiences, and, more specifically, they may ask you what you have learned from these experiences.

Let's take a look at an example of an elective leadership position, outside of medical-school applications, where you may also be asked about your leadership roles and experiences. For example, when applying for a job, especially management-level employment, you might be asked to fill out some forms and attend an interview.

Paramount on the interviewer's to-do list is usually a series of questions to ascertain leadership qualities in the applicant. This series of questions is designed to help identify the candidates who have the ability to find the time to learn about, work with, and strengthen the weakest link in any chain of people whom they might have to work with or for whom they might become responsible.

In addition, many employment interviewers search for a candidate who has the gift of being able to recognize the unique qualities and skills in colleagues and subordinates that they could enlist to achieve success in working toward a common goal. Equally important, the interviewer is looking for the management (leadership) candidate who will inspire others to follow their dreams—as grandiose or as trivial as they may seem at the time.

Frequently, the interviewer will have a list of questions that are designed to find a leader among leaders. They are looking for an individual who is a confident leader and recognizes the strengths of each of the individuals that he or she is working with as standouts in their own right. They are seeking a person who is able to inspire each individual to do what is needed, as a team, to get the task done. Hmm, sounds like they might be looking for a first-round draft pick for the NFL.

Being able to assume leadership in nonelective circumstances (read: crises and/or emergencies) often requires a different skill set. In high-stress or crisis situations, this set of leadership skills would include the ability to calmly and steadfastly restore order, establish command of the situation, whatever it may be, and be able to enlist others to assist in and carry out the numerous tasks necessary to navigate through the particular crisis or emergency.

These types of leadership skills are seen time and time again in history. Prominent examples include Arthur Wellesley, Napoleon Bonaparte, Alexander the Great, and Julius Caesar. Their battle-honed leadership skills consistently served them well and led to new positions for each of them in governing their respective domains.

Crisis and emergency leadership skills are also prominently seen in the business world. We see examples on the news and in the movies. In fact, Donald Trump created a successful television series, *The Apprentice*, in which he created a business crisis each week for famous participants to duke it out and assume the leadership role. Those who weren't successful were fired by Trump.

As a doctor you will be required to be a leader on many levels. You will be expected to be a leader in both elective circumstances and nonelective circumstances. In many communities, doctors are also looked up to as pillars of their social community and are expected to be role models for others, young and old.

The postgraduate medical education system, also called residency, is the next step after medical school. Residency is designed to teach not only refinement of skills and knowledge but also how to lead. Each resident, at each level of residency, is responsible for the decisions and actions as well as the results, good or bad, of the residents and medical students on their service. In other words, a chief resident is responsible for the decisions, actions, and results of the medical students, PGY-1 (postgraduate year 1), PGY-2, PGY-3, PGY-4, and so on who are on his or her service. That is a lot of responsibility when you stop and think about it. The decisions, actions, and results that I am talking about involve the health care and well-being of actual living patients.

A great deal of the success or failure at each PGY level is determined by the development, or lack thereof, of leadership skills.

By now, you should get the picture as to why medical-school admissions committees put a lot of emphasis on the medical-school applicant's leadership qualities and demonstration of these skills.

How do you demonstrate personal leadership qualities and skills, criteria that are often used to evaluate and separate the best among the best?

You should constantly look for opportunities for leadership. They exist all around you. Start with what you are interested in. This is always the tree that bears the most fruit. After all, we do best with what we are most interested in. Pursuing our passions as leaders makes it all the more wonderful.

We are most at ease with that which we are familiar with, that in which we are secure in our understanding, and that in which we are confident in our abilities. These, by the way, are three characteristics that we see in effective leaders.

If you are able to identify with and associate these three characteristics with an activity that you like, then you have a real winner. For example, if you enjoy...let's see...pre-Colombian jade carvings, you can make this a golden opportunity. You can start off by researching a group that is already on campus, attending its regular meetings, becoming active in the group, volunteering for the annual fundraiser, and unswervingly working your way up through the ranks to become an officer and leader.

Seriously, you might find it a little easier to find and join the debate club, chess club, a cultural club, youth club, religious club, or political club and apply the same principles. Other opportunities abound. The glee club and orchestra will often have many levels of opportunity to demonstrate leadership skills.

And of course there is the wide-open category of sports and cheerleading. Sports and cheerleading lend themselves naturally to the development and implementation of leadership skills. Participation over a period of years goes a long way in demonstrating consistency in a task. Work with a mentor or a coach. He or she can really teach you and help you develop your leadership skills. And if you really work at it and hone your skills, it will be a huge feather in your cap to be elected or named captain or cocaptain of your squad or team.

I have seen numerous occasions when an applicant had decent grades and average MCATs, but consistent participation on a team and having been a captain or cocaptain (demonstration of strong leadership skills) is what made the difference in acceptance to medical school.

You can also demonstrate leadership in off-campus activities. Working in the community, in various social programs, lends itself very well to this goal. And you get to help out people in need at the same time. How great is that?

Where to start? Well, how about programs that already exist? For example, getting involved in a program such as Habitat for Humanity is a good place to begin. As you consistently work to help others and become an integral part or the Habitat team, you can practice your leadership skills, newly acquired or otherwise, and eventually become a team leader. How about working your way up through the rank and file at a local soup kitchen or youth center?

You might be thinking, "None of these suggestions works for me. What should I do?"

Well...get ready for the best and most exciting suggestion of all. Ready? Drum roll...wait for it...

Start your own group!

And guess what? By starting your own club, group, society, or team and populating it, you automatically are its leader. How about that? But please make sure that it is truly an organization that is doing something positive and helpful for your school or local community. Remember the admonition from earlier in this chapter.

When I first established my surgical practice in sunny South Florida, it quickly became evident that there was an overwhelming need for a professional society in my specialty for social, ethical, professional, and educational reasons. Unfortunately, in later years, we had to add political reasons to the list. But that's a story for another day. Well, anyhow, there was no such professional society in our county.

One of my colleagues and I formed the society, created the bylaws, and populated it. He was senior and became the first president, and I became the first vice-president. And, as it happened, I became the second president. This led to many more leadership positions for me over the years. So the point is, there was an absence, a need, and a willing population—and then, voilà, instant leadership. Go on, give it a try.

There are students at my university who have formed cultural dance groups, acting groups, student interest groups, intramural sports teams, and the list goes on. So go ahead and ask yourself, "What can I do? How can I become a leader?"

As the popular saying goes, "Just Do It."

10. Research

Many students are hung up on the concept of research. The pre-medical student, in particular, is a victim of the "research mentality"—and for good reason.

The research mentality is a carry-over from a particular graduate school philosophy—or, more accurately, a graduate school requirement. Graduate students, including master's thesis students and PhD students, are required to publish their research in order to fulfill the requirements to graduate. The faculty members are also required to publish their research to bolster their faculty standing and the prestige of their institution. But, the faculty has the added burden to publish their research for a very simple reason.

They are fully aware that they must "publish or perish."

Publishing, with its inherent grant money, is a major source of funds for supporting faculty, staff, students, equipment, and facilities at a great many institutions.

There are many medical schools that are research oriented. Undergraduates who want to attend these particular research-oriented medical schools would do well to already have multiple published research projects under their belts. These published projects can include poster presentations, abstracts, and/or articles in significant peer-reviewed journals as primary investigator (PI) or as one of multiple authors.

Over the past many decades, there has been the impression that having been actively involved in research is a necessity to bolster and strengthen a medical-school application.

For a growing number of medical schools today, the desirability of premedical applicants who have participated in and published their research has been in a downhill slide of declining importance. Keep in mind that there are still plenty of medical schools that encourage student research. By viewing individual medical-school program descriptions and requirements, you will be able to determine which medical schools are best suited for you.

Although having a publication or publications does look good listed on your medical-school application, it in no way carries the same weight or importance that having a publication did up until a few short years ago.

With the current shortage of physicians in America, the pendulum has swung in the other direction. Every year, more and more medical schools are shifting their emphasis to clinical education and patient focus. More and more medical schools are introducing and emphasizing to medical students the importance of clinical medicine from the get-go, at the very start—day one of the first year of medical school. Of course, medical-school education is not entirely clinically based. There is still plenty of formal and traditional classroom and small-group work, which is integrated with, and supports, the clinical education that is being offered to medical students.

Medical schools are also shifting a lot of emphasis to the study of social sciences. The relationships between doctors, nurses, social workers, allied health workers, and, most importantly, patients are in a dynamic state of overhaul.

The MCAT (Medical College Admission Test) reflects this shift in medical-school emphasis with an entirely new section that tests one's knowledge and application of the social sciences, including sociology and psychology. Individual medical schools have different philosophies and will put emphasis on the qualities and experiences they find most desirous for the selection of medical-school applicants whom they believe will be the best fit.

Research, although a plus, is being deemphasized by many medical schools. Research experience is a major plus for those medical schools that emphasize research within their curriculums. If you choose to do research to include on your medical-school application, there are a few different ways to go about it.

The quickest, easiest pathway to finding interesting (and doable) research projects is to look on the bulletin board, electronic or otherwise, of the various subdivisions of your university's science department. Science departments are always looking for grunts, gophers ("go fors"), or lab rats. And that is exactly what you will be.

More than likely you will be someone who is just a body to be used to clean up a mess or make a donut and coffee run. You really won't get anything truly meaningful out of this experience. But this position will allow you to fill in the blank of your AMCAS (American Medical College Application Service) application showing that you did research.

Why stop there? You can discuss your research in depth at your interview, right? Unfortunately, or should I say fortunately, this type of "research" (nonresearch) is easily identified and picked up by the admissions committee, particularly at the interview, as nonsensical and totally without merit or value.

If you decide that you want to and are going to do research, you might as well make it a positive experience that will not only enhance your medical-school application but also actually teach you something about research and, at the same time, enhance your knowledge of whatever subject you choose to research. You might consider talking with a few of your professors or more communicative teaching assistants (TAs) about their research and how you might fit in as a member of the teams. A truthful, heartfelt discussion will go a long way toward finding a comfortable fit and avoiding a catastrophe.

If you want to be savvy, I would suggest that you begin early, during your sophomore year of college, so that your research is well underway by the time you put together your medical-school application. Working with a professor or TA (teaching assistant), you can develop your own research project. Wow, now that's exciting!

Look at the world and think about how you might try to answer some fundamental question, and actually do it. What a display of creativity, consistency, and commitment that would be. What admissions committee wouldn't be all over that?

There is another option that I would venture to suggest to you. It is the option with the most bang for your buck, the one that will have a positive impact on your application, the one in which you will be able to demonstrate and accomplish two of the major objectives of your medical-school application; and it is also the research option that will be the most fun and usually the most rewarding, especially for young medical-school applicants. What am I talking about?

The answer is clinical research.

In almost every institution of medical education, as well as major (and not-so-major) hospitals and private practices across the country, there are clinical research projects underway. Some of these projects are prospective and have a great need for someone like you to collect and compile data. Or, with a little proper training, you can learn to analyze data.

Think about it. The opportunities are endless: drug therapy studies, surgical outcome studies, medical device studies, epidemiological studies, case management studies, and the list goes on and on. With the use of e-mail and an effective Google search, you will be able to avoid an overwhelming number of letters, phone calls, and personal visits. This gives a whole new meaning to "let your fingers do the walking."

I have previously mentioned that with clinical research, you will be able to accomplish two of the major objectives of your medical-school application, and you will. You will be doing research, plus you will be exposed to numerous patient contact hours. How cool is that? Very cool!

It is also very helpful—let me rephrase that—it is *imperative* that you are conversant in the subject of your research. This is especially true at the time of your interview! It is important to be able to explain the "significance of 6-glutathione alpha reductase in the redox reaction of gamma amino aloha acid and its significance in peroxide synthesis."

Will your interviewer have any idea of what you are talking about? If you are doing bench research, make sure you can dumb it down quite a few notches. On the other hand, if you are involved in clinical research, you will have to understand it thoroughly and be entirely conversant in every aspect of your research project.

More than likely your interviewer will be conversant on the subject of your research because he or she read your application the day before your interview and then studied the topic of your research in great detail. Your interviewer may even be able to ask you intelligent and apropos questions on the subject of your research. *So be well prepared.* Practice presenting the main theme and ideas of your research to friends and family, especially to those who know nothing about the subject or topic of your research.

You want to be able to explain your research in layman's terms so that anyone at any time will understand you. This is especially important if your interviewer is a nonscientist or someone who is not research based. You want to make it easy for your interviewer to understand your work and the importance of it. Otherwise, you risk the chance that your interviewer will just gloss over your work.

If you have done your research solely to add to the list of achievements on your medical-school application, you can see the ramifications of having missed the golden opportunity at your interview for you to help your interviewer to understand and comment on your research in their postinterview report.

If you have done your research because you truly wanted to and dedicated your time and efforts with passion, then you lost the moment to demonstrate to your interviewer your creativity, consistency, and commitment. But all is not lost. These "three Cs" will have been noted from your brief description in the activities section of your medical-school application.

You should set a time limit to your explanation. Develop and practice a one-minute, sound-bite version as well as a five-minute, complete explanation.

If you encounter an interviewer who has no knowledge of your subject and is disinterested in your research, then the one-minute version will be perfect. Any longer than that, and your explanation will turn your interviewer off and actually work against you. This type of interviewer really doesn't care the slightest bit about your research but will more than likely be smart enough to follow your *brief* explanation. He or she will really be listening to verify that you actually did the research, and beyond that, he or she won't care.

Please don't let me make a complete cynic out of you. Remember, your research played a role in getting you to the interview in the first place.

Now for those interviewers who are truly interested in you and who you really are, and for those interviewers who do understand and appreciate your research, the five-minute version will come in handy.

Take your time and tell your story, smartly. Tell a complete story with a beginning, middle, and ending that is clear and concise. Build it up, drag it out a little, glorify in the results, draw diagrams, draw little squiggles, and build to a crescendo with your magnificent conclusions. After all, you will be receiving a Nobel Prize—one day—for the fruits of your labor.

If you can find out if the medical schools that you are applying to have branded themselves in a particular area, such as geriatrics or public health, then you can also enhance your cache if you are clever.

Obviously, when you began your particular research project, there was no way you would have known the standout specialties and areas of enhanced concentration of the medical schools that you would be applying to months or years later.

However, if you have an idea about which medical schools you will be applying to—or, better yet, if you know the top two or three choices of medical schools you will be applying to—then you can use this knowledge to your advantage.

Start or join a research project in a field that is consistent with the standout specialties and areas of enhanced concentration of the medical school(s) that you will be applying to. If that is not an option for you, you need not worry about it. As you will be wisely applying to numerous medical schools, the odds are highly in your favor that if you are involved in clinical research in subjects that are currently "hot items," such as geriatrics, rural medicine, and public health, you will be in sync with the interests of many medical-school programs.

You will certainly catch the attention of the admissions-committee member(s) who first evaluates your application, and this will greatly increase the likelihood of your being invited for an interview at that particular institution.

If you have no idea about the areas of focus for the medical schools that you are applying to (I sincerely hope that you did your homework on this in advance of applying), but find out at the interview-day introduction and orientation that your research project might just fit into their interests, then sit back, reflect, and work it.

Show your interviewer how your interests and the interests of this particular medical school are a natural fit (much more on this in the chapter "The Interview").

If you preach to the choir, it will listen!

11. The Fire Hydrant

You might be asking yourself, "Why is he including a chapter titled 'The Fire Hydrant' in the middle of a book on getting into medical school?"

And I would reply, "That is a very good question."

The fire hydrant—what a great concept.

I have included in this book many odd, different, interesting, and helpful concepts. We have talked about the need to "stop studying for exams." We have discussed planting a seed and waiting for a tree bearing fruit to grow from it. We enjoyed the conversation about a vessel with a liquid in it that was an exercise in how to think out of the box. Later in this book, we will talk about creating, writing, directing, and starring in your own movie.

So why are we talking about a fire hydrant?

The concept of the fire hydrant is a concept that was just recently introduced to me by one of my medical students. Considering that I am always open to new ideas and perceptions, I readily understood what she was saying to me. It did take a few minutes for me to realize how deep the fire-hydrant analogy really was.

We are often exposed to new concepts and new ways to look at things. As long as our minds are open, we can absorb, evaluate, synthesize, organize, recall, and apply new concepts. But we can't receive new thoughts and concepts unless we open our minds to such wonderful gifts. In actuality, we are constantly exposed to new concepts. To receive these incredible gifts, we must have our "receiver" turned on. If we live on a narrow path, one where we are excessively concentrating only on that which is directly in front of our noses, then we miss out on all the signals that are trying to break through and stimulate our receivers.

Too many of us use one sense at a time. If we are eating, we are consumed with taste. If we are listening to music, we might be distracted from other tasks. The best example of this, or perhaps I should say the worst example, is the evidenced-based data that clearly demonstrates the horrific increase in traffic accidents and fatalities associated with cell phone use—and I am not referring only to texting—and talking while driving.

Many of you reading this book are familiar with how the human brain works. For those of you who are not familiar with this absolutely amazing "ground zero" of our body functions, I will give you a short-and-sweet review.

The human brain is an organ with the consistency of Jell-O that is enclosed within a dense, hard container called the skull. The brain consists of one hundred billion neurons (nerve cells), give or take a few billion. These special nerve cells are surrounded by fat and connective tissue, and they have a rich blood supply. In fact, the human body will sacrifice blood from all other areas of the body in order to ensure an adequate blood supply to the brain. Also, to act as a shock absorber and to protect it against trauma, concussions, and tissue destruction, the brain is surrounded by a few membranes and a layer of cerebrospinal fluid.

Within the brain, as I mentioned a little earlier, there are billions of neurons. These neurons, interacting with each other 24-7, enable all of our life processes to take place. The brain controls breathing and heart rate. The brain regulates blood pressure and how fast we can run. The brain interprets what we see, hear, smell, taste, and touch. But really, how does the brain do all of this? How does the brain work?

Conventional science tells us that all of the brain's functions are basically carried out by constant, continuous chemical reactions in all sorts of feedback loops. There is so much evidence to support this that there really is no argument. But there is a whole other unexplored aspect of the brain. We see much evidence of this activity around us, and yet we have little to no understanding of it. Science shows us that bats, whales, porpoises, and shrews are able to utilize echolocation—sonar. How do they do it? How do they produce sound waves from inside their brains and then receive and interpret them? Scientists are studying this phenomenon to find the answers. Back in the 1960s, during the Apollo program, Norman Mailer, who was a very famous author at the time, set up some experiments with some of the astronauts. I was fortunate enough to see some of the interviews between Norman Mailer and the astronauts. The astronauts clearly and succinctly discussed their experience of being able to communicate with each other with thought, not using words. I find it intriguing that after these interviews, the whole project was dropped, and nothing was ever said or published again on these particular experiments.

The point of this entire discussion is to open your mind to how seemingly limitless the human brain is in its ability to perform at levels that we are just beginning to scratch the surface of understanding.

In Rhonda Byrne's book *The Secret*, she anecdotally describes many examples of thought being transformed into results. In the book *The Passion Test*, authors Janet and Chris Atwood actually provide a blueprint on how to do it. Yes, you read that right. They teach you how to define your passions and achieve them by putting the right signals out and, just as importantly, how to receive the responses.

Maybe we are more like bats, whales, porpoises, and shrews than we realize.

How does this relate to you, the medical-school applicant, and what does this have to do with fire hydrants? Let us see.

The human brain is incredible. It truly is a masterful example of the ultimate multitasker. It is also the penultimate example of one of the corollaries of the Peter Principle: "The work expands to fill the time allotted to it." Or, in better words, "If you want something done, give it to a busy person."

In the case of medical students, and paraphrasing quite liberally, no matter how much work and studying you demand of medical students, they will get it done.

One of the most difficult things for high-school graduates to get a handle on when they first attend college is the tremendous increase in workload that they are faced with in class and in additional homework. Somehow most make it and graduate college. The most difficult obstacle that college graduates in the first few months of medical school are challenged with is the even greater increase in classwork and homework. And I am talking about a whole magnitude greater than college. There isn't just a lot of stuff to learn; there is also an abundance of clinical work and a large amount of time needed to prepare presentations.

You can easily see that all of this work and "stuff" can, and does, become overwhelming—and very quickly.

It is a true task to make it all happen. It is a Herculean task to make it all work for you and in such a way that you are not just spinning your wheels.

The two greatest tools to make it all happen and work for you are:

1. the "fire hydrant," which I will get to, momentarily, and
2. the principles that I cover in detail in the chapter titled "You Have Nothing to Fear but Fear Itself."

Let's first discuss the latter briefly. When faced with any large obstacle or challenge, most of us will develop a feeling of self-doubt or of being overwhelmed. This is particularly true for marathoners and mountain climbers.

Many, if not most, marathoners view any particular marathon, and especially the one they are about to start, not as a 26.2-mile race but rather as a series of small races tacked onto each other. They see four 5K races (3.1 miles each) followed by a final 10K race (6.2 miles). In other words, they break down the large, daunting task into a series of smaller, less scary blocks. They focus on each block individually, and when one block is finished, they easily move on to the next block, and so forth. Each block is seen individually and is easier to complete. Add all of the blocks together, and you finish the structure—or in this case, the marathon.

In the chapter titled "You Have Nothing to Fear but Fear Itself," I discuss the plight of some inexperienced mountain climbers—myself among them—and how a very experienced mountaineer, "Mr. Everest," helped them to overcome their group fear and feelings of being overwhelmed by the task set before them—climbing a very large mountain. The bottom line was that each climber only had to decide to take the first step. And then another. And then another. Eventually they would all arrive at the top of the mountain. And that is exactly how it is for all mountain climbers.

This is exactly how it is for new medical students faced with an incredible load of work and studying. My students have learned, as did I when I was a medical student, that it works best to chip away at the block a little piece at a time.

Medical students learn to become superb time managers in order to survive. In fact, it is the only way for them to survive. Part of becoming an excellent, successful doctor is to become an excellent, successful time manager.

The good news is that it all starts right in the first year of medical school.

Most medical schools will go easy on new students for the first week or so. Then the onslaught begins. Some students will ease into the work, and other students will let it pile up. The mellow students will let things happen as they happen. The "gunners" will continue their premed ethic and do whatever it takes to make themselves look better than the rest of their classmates (take heart in knowing that modifying this type of gunner behavior is the goal of the medical education office and the faculty at medical schools) and will adopt a take-no-prisoners approach to everything.

I always wondered how today's premedical students and medical students were able to keep up with the workload expected of them. The largest component of the workload is the gargantuan amount of studying and education-related tasks. Yes, I was faced with the same issues when I was a premed and medical student. But it just seems like there is so much more expected of students today.

I remember my first day of orientation at the George Washington University School of Medicine when one of the deans stated, "All of the information that a doctor could acquire and study during his entire lifetime in the days of our first president, George Washington, you will acquire and be responsible for knowing in one week." That was like a kick in the head.

Today I could say to medical-school applicants and medical students, "All of the information that I learned just a couple of decades ago to become a successful and excellent doctor, you will have to learn in a couple of months."

The amount of knowledge and technical advancements that have been achieved in the last few decades exceeds the sum of all knowledge and technical advancement of the last few thousand years of human civilization.

How does today's student keep up? How does today's student learn it all?

This leads perfectly into our discussion of the fire hydrant.

Over the many years that I have been teaching interns, residents, and medical students, I have continually asked myself, "How do they do it?" The fact that I already went through it never entered my mind because, as I explained above, the amount of work and the time commitment has skyrocketed.

Sure, it was easy for me to think about how "work expands to fill the time allotted to it," but I knew very well that "time does not expand to fulfill the work demanded of it." It wasn't until I entered into my role as an admissions-committee member that I learned the answer. During the course of hundreds of medical-school interviews, I have learned a lot about people. I also have learned a lot of fascinating information, and not all of it was medically related. In fact, the most interesting conversations were philosophical, including great discussions about Gandhi, Malthus, Descartes, Curious George, the Little Engine That Could, and quite a few others.

I was totally surprised, after so many years seeking an answer to this big question, that it was a student in her first week of medical school, in orientation, who was the agent of delivery to me—and now to you—of such an incredibly important, yet elegantly simple answer to the question that remained so annoyingly in the forefront of my thinking. "How do you make the time expand to fit the volume of work demanded?" I find that it is not only a simple and clever answer, but it also serves as a wonderful teaching aid and an absolute must for all students to think about and visualize.

Ready? Well, here it is in all of its simplistic ingenuity.

Up until now, up until this point in your scholastic life, you have been drinking from a water fountain. Now, you are being forced to drink from a fire hydrant.

"Say what?"

Up until now, your education, and life in general, has come to you in small, easily digested pieces. In keeping with the theme of this conversation, it would be more appropriate for me to say that your education has been coming to you in a slow, constant flow and that you have absorbed all of it with small, continuous sips.

Think of it this way. Previously, you were drinking from the slow, easy laminar flow of a water fountain. All that you had to do was press the button, and the water was delivered to you in a slow, easy flow, from which it was easy to swallow all of it, without spilling a drop. In fact, you probably had the capacity to drink and absorb more but felt no need to do so. You probably just wanted to sip away at your own easy pace, just enough to slake your thirst of immediate needs.

And then everything changed.

The water fountain has become a fire hydrant. Rather than slow, easy sipping, you are getting inundated with stuff. Today you can't take your time and sip. You have to put in your entire face, your entire head, and swallow as much water as you can gulp down. You are fully aware that you can't swallow all of it, but you swallow as much as you can. The key is to swallow and absorb the central core. With time you can, and will, adapt to the increased flow of demands.

Fortunately, the system understands this and will recapture for you the excess and recirculate it for you again and again. In the world of medical education, repetition (and still more repetition) is called residency. Every day, week after week, year after year, you keep seeing the same stuff in different forms and guises. With enough repetition, it eventually becomes a part of your soul, your very being. This is one of the reasons that the process to become a doctor is so long and time-consuming.

In the medical and surgical specialties that are technique dependent and physically hands-on, such as the surgical specialties and interventional medical specialties, there is a time-tested method by which they guarantee that you learn the material and gather sufficient knowledge. It is best summed up in an old and very apropos adage: "See one, do one, teach one," or, paraphrasing liberally, see many, do many, teach many.

It really boils down to repetition leading to awareness, absorption, assimilation, and application. Then you get to teach it to somebody else. After all, teaching others is an extremely strong incentive to thoroughly learn any subject and really understand it.

The idea is to expose you to as much as possible—the fire hydrant—so that you can get the big picture in one big dose. Some people can take bigger gulps, and others swallow a lot faster. In the short run, you are examined and graded on your retention and ability to apply what you swallowed for any particular course.

No one expects you to remember it all. You can only swallow as much as you can gulp down *and* retain. And you can only take one gulp at a time. There is a lot that misses your mouth, and you can't recover it. Then you can only look forlornly at it as it slides down the drain. Don't be upset. You will see it over and over again, and you will be a terrific doctor.

Up until now, just about all that you have had to learn at school, and in life in general, has been presented to you in an organized, linear fashion. Kindergarten through twelfth grade and college are purposely designed to be presented in a slow, ponderous fashion. Educators at this level want to be sure that the population receives a general education. And for the most part, the system works.

But you are not average, and you never will be. You require more education, and the medical system will require more of you. Your future career and your future patients will make incredible demands of you. You will be ready. Drinking from the fire hydrant is preparing you every single time that you take a gulp.

Of course, life might throw a curveball here and there, and things might get a bit chaotic from time to time. Catastrophes such as the great life stressors—birth, marriage, being fired, a new job, divorce, bad grades (I added that one in there—after all, you are a student), illness, and death—can also interrupt life, your education, and your career.

Right now, at this very moment in time, many of you are preparing yourselves and doing everything conceivable in your power to get accepted into medical school.

When you combine the life stressors that you might be experiencing with the markedly increased difficulty and time commitment of upper-level courses, an increasingly demanding schedule, MCAT prep, medical volunteerism, community service, research, and visiting and interviewing at medical schools, you find that your previously organized, time-managed life is becoming totally random and chaotic. Let's not forget about all of the studying, too.

It seems that life in general has changed. It wasn't too long ago that we lived in a "nuclear family." All you had to do was get up in the morning; eat breakfast with your family; go to school; go home; fit in your homework before and after the dinner you would have with your family; and then have a little free time to read, watch TV, or whatever. Now we live in a global community thanks to computers, the Internet, and all of the offshoots.

Today you probably spend hours on the computer playing *Words with Friends* with virtual friends in Singapore, *Flappy Bird* with virtual friends in Portugal, or texting for hours with your classmates. How much time do you spend on your iPhone or iPad? Like it or not, you are in the fire-hydrant generation.

When I was a younger student—I am still a student—my generation demanded silence while studying. We would bury ourselves in a study hall, library, dorm room (ha-ha, not too quiet), or apartment.

Today, it just ain't so. I used to get on my son's case about all of the distractions going on around him while he was studying. I was the study police. Now that I have seen the results of his "megatasking," not multitasking, I have become an advocate of a laissez-faire study police policy. He is a straight-A student and a student leader at his school. His younger sister is following his example with great success.

There you have it. My generation, and previous generations, lived and learned in a water-fountain fashion. Our world was linear, and we were able to live and learn at a slower pace with occasional bursts of chaos and frenzy. You live in a world of constant input, with an unceasing multimedia bombardment of information. You live in a world of exponential change. The information highway keeps growing, and the speed limit increases with every passing day. You are from the fire-hydrant generation. As long as it continues to be successful, without burnout, who am I to judge?

12. Dreams—Don't Let Them Take Them Away

To help drive home the point of this important chapter, I would like to tell you a short story.

Ever since I was a little boy, like every little boy and girl, I had dreams. I had dreams of being a cowboy. Being a fireman sure did seem like a great idea. Wow, I wanted to be an astronaut. But even before I wanted to be a doctor, which I decided I wanted to be when I was eight, I really wanted to become a marine biologist and under-sea explorer.

Life was a little different "back in the day." It was a very different world then. We didn't have any of the amazing diversions that families and kids have today. I used to laugh when my mom would tell me about her childhood and how her family would gather each evening after dinner and listen to the radio, read, or play cards.

It was a little more interesting for families of my day. We had black and white and then color television. So instead of sitting around the radio, reading and playing cards, my generation would sit and stare at one of seven television stations. Every Sunday night we would especially hurry through dinner to watch "Sunday television." Sunday was a family night, and we would all zone out and transport ourselves to other worlds and incredible adventures. It is basically the same idea, in a very low-tech version, as happens with today's children. Only my children escape into their Xbox or PlayStation.

Well, anyway, I would run off a little earlier so that I could escape into the *Wonderful World of Disney*. Every week there was a different fantastic adventure. The theme would vary over a four-week period: the old frontier, battling evil knights and witches, outer space and beyond, or some faraway kingdom on a pirate ship. Mr. Disney sure had a great concept. It is amazing, and truly wonderful, that this idea still thrills children today and brings them together from all over the world to experience amazing adventures and fantasies at Disneyland and Disney World.

Well, once again I digressed. After the *Wonderful World of Disney*, the whole family would watch Ed Sullivan and his amazing variety show. This is the same show that introduced the Beatles and the Rolling Stones to the United States.

Every few months, this Sunday night tradition would be interrupted. Perhaps it would be better to say it was exponentially enhanced. After a week of off-the-charts TV advertising and buildup, Sunday night would be filled with what for me was the most exquisite, wonderful, otherworldly display of pure freedom, color, and emotion. I am referring to the landmark programming called *The Undersea World of Jacques Cousteau*.

Cousteau, his sons, and his crew would present their world. It was a brave, exciting, and foreign world. It was an incredible world of undersea exploration, which was a place more foreign and otherworldly than outer space (this was all happening during the cold war and the race to space with the Soviet Union). All the while, the Cousteaus interspersed their message of conservationism and ecological preservation. It was this beautiful, foreign, and exciting world that I was enthralled with, as were thousands of children who would religiously watch this special presentation whenever it was scheduled on this major network channel. Yes, there was a world before cable television.

The most spectacular aspect of this world of Jacques Cousteau was that, in addition to all of the beauty, social consciousness, and exploration, he got to do it from the most technologically advanced marine exploratory platform of its day. He lived, worked, played, explored, and educated from his beautiful, majestic, sanguine, and lovely *Calypso*. She was a beautiful ship, and she was named after Calypso, the siren of Homer's *Odyssey*. As told by Homer, Calypso would capture the heart of any sailor who viewed her. From the moment when I first saw her, albeit on television, I was smitten. I bought and read all of Jacques Cousteau's artistically worded and illustrated books. They were truly beautiful. Each page was adorned with magnificent underwater photographs. The book was full of glossy, magazine-quality pages with the most beautiful photographs and writing, accentuating the Cousteau message. I lived and dreamed of *Calypso* and her explorations to the exotic corners of the world. I knew that I had to be part of it, part of her adventure, and a part of her history.

Of course, when I got a little older, I trained hard and earned my scuba certification. This was back when certification numbers were still in the hundreds and when we did not have pressure gages, buoyancy compensation, or other safety devices. I would dive as often as I could on vacations and summers off from my studies at the university and during the years of preparation to apply to medical school.

Over the years I maintained my love for *Calypso* and the amazing explorations being done by Jacques Cousteau and the crew. And then it happened: the first link was solidly forged in the chain to bring me to her, to *Calypso*. I was accepted to medical school at the George Washington University School of Medicine, right in our nation's capital. I knew that if I continued to dedicate myself to my lessons in medicine and continued to study the oceans, then I would somehow find a way to make it to *Calypso*.

And then the second seismic event occurred. It was during my second year of medical school at GW that I learned that my idol, Jacques Cousteau, was coming to Washington, DC, to present his work in a spectacular lecture and presentation, open to the public. Thankfully, it was in the evening after classes.

The venue was jammed, shoulder to shoulder, with thousands of interested people. His presentation was as amazing and fascinating as I had imagined it would be. It was as mesmerizing as when I was growing up and watching Cousteau and *Calypso* on TV. I waited until the very end of the lecture and until the question and answer period was over. I waited until almost everyone had filed out of the auditorium. And then I was ready to forge the next link in the chain to *Calypso*.

I approached Jacques Cousteau; *the* Jacques Cousteau. He was my lifelong hero and the modern explorer and scientist who sailed *Calypso*. He looked at me with his light-blue, knowing eyes. I stepped up to him, and I felt my heart pounding so hard in my chest that I thought it would rip right out of me. With a large smile on my face, I began to tell him of my dream. I told him of all the years I'd had this dream. I went on to explain, "I graduated from The George Washington University with a bachelor's of science in zoology, and now I am in my second year of medical school. When I earn my degree in medicine, I would like to volunteer and contribute my time and knowledge to working with you on *Calypso*."

The hammer was about to strike the anvil; the next link was about to be forged. But little did I expect how the hammer would be wielded. He looked me right in the eyes and said, "Take you? Why? We are serious in what we do. Take you, ha." He then promptly turned his back and walked away. The hammer came down and smashed the chain.

At that moment, at that very moment, I was crushed. My plan was shattered. I couldn't believe it. "This didn't just happen. Is this a dream? It just can't be."

Denial.

My dream—he took it away!

Then for the next few years, I seethed in anger and disappointment. I strongly felt that Cousteau was a self-centered, self-aggrandizing, and arrogant man. Or so I thought, at that particular time, and denied any other possible alternative or reason for the episode (denial). I reasoned that he must be mean and quite nasty to everyone (anger). I then went through a period of questioning myself and making deals and promises to God that if I could do good deeds (which I should have been doing anyway) or give up the physical and worldly pleasures of life (monastic life is not very stylish in the United States), then I should easily be gifted with a call by Jacques Cousteau asking me to come aboard and work with him on the *Calypso* (bargaining). I then became upset, sad, and disheartened. My dream was gone. He had taken my dream away (depression). What was I going to do? I had always dreamed of being the doctor aboard *Calypso*. When I seriously analyzed my situation, I came up with some cogent and obvious answers (acceptance).

I truly did think about and kept asking myself, "What really is my dream?" What was it that I had truly visualized as my future, my calling? What was it that I had been dedicating myself to all along? What was it that I had worked so hard to achieve and never stopped focusing on? Duh! The answer had been in front of me all along and was so clear and obvious.

My true, primary dream was to become a doctor, and to become the best doctor that I could possibly be.

Jacques Cousteau was a gift—a small blip, a little bit of chaos in my life to help me transform and grow into the strong, dedicated doctor I was destined to become. Since that sentinel event in Washington, DC, I have often wondered about the true nature of my encounter with Jacques Cousteau. I have often wondered if his denial of my dream was the only purpose for our encounter, or if, alternatively, Mr. Cousteau was totally aware, at the time of what he denied me and why he was denying it. Today, decades later, I do not see the event as I did then. It actually wasn't a denial but rather an invitation for personal growth. I now see that I was just too immature and blind to see how miraculous the universe is in putting us in a specific place, at a specific time, so that we can be present at the sentinel transition points in our lives.

Throughout your lifetime, opportunities will be placed in your path on a regular basis. These opportunities will be disguised in many forms. Be prepared to be knocked around a little. Be ready to face frustrations and blockages. The trick is to realize that every time chaos enters your life, it is an opportunity for you to grow and to exceed yourself. Each wall gives you the gift of growth, new wisdom, and strength to progress forward to greater excellence.

Before I move forward to other examples of "dream taking," let me ask you a question. Did you recognize within the ending of the above short story the utilization and interpretation of the theory of the five stages of grief? This theory is the centerpiece of the brilliant and ground-breaking book *On Death and Dying*, written by Elizabeth Kübler-Ross in 1969. Her work is applicable to so many circumstances and situations in life.

The key is to recognize when you are right dead-center in the middle of it. The key is to recognize for yourself that you are experiencing one of the five stages at the time that you are actually experiencing the stage. If you are aware that you are in the middle of the process, it will help make difficult times less difficult. This recognition, and being patient with each stage, will make for much smoother sailing through any time of great angst. Recognizing that you are in one of the five stages will make it much easier for you to open the door, step through, and then enter the path of the next stage.

As human beings we all have times of grief, sorrow, and disappointment. Passing through the five stages of grief keeps us going and helps us to continue pursuing our dreams. Do yourself a huge favor and read Kübler-Ross.

One of the benefits that almost all universities in the United States make available to premedical students is the premedical advisor. They come in many forms, shapes, and sizes. Obviously, the shape and size don't matter. The form is of utmost importance.

At most universities, the premedical advisors are often the teachers, instructors, or professors who are employees of universities and colleges. Classically, teachers, instructors, and professors are underpaid and overworked. However, in the socioeconomic climate of the last few years in the United States, there have been ever-worsening budget constraints for private and state-funded schools.

University professors already have a full schedule and workload. Their assignments of responsibility are filled to overflowing with their teaching, administrative, and research obligations. Add to that budget constraints and cutbacks, and you can readily see that the load continues to increase for each professor. These are the lucky ones. Those not so lucky have lost their jobs.

Consider this environment and the stress that each of the surviving professors has to live and work with every day, and then you walk in, asking for advice and taking up more of the professor's time. Again, I ask you to visualize the atmosphere of stress that your teacher (and advisor) is working under, and then you walk in, giving him or her additional work and taking up his or her valuable time.

I truly believe that for the majority of student advisors, and particularly premedical advisors, their intentions are good, and they want to do the very best for you. Premedical student advisors are special advisors in that they are dealing with the cream of the crop of college students. Not only are premed advisors trying to help you get the highest grades possible, they are also trying to give you the best advice about your future life choices.

Because they are already so overwhelmed and have multiple responsibilities for so many obligations, however, their ability to advise you might suffer, and it may not take precedence for them.

I already stated, and want to emphatically repeat, that the majority of premedical advisors are excellent, responsible, and professional advisors.

And then there are those who aren't excellent, responsible, or professional advisors. Unfortunately, you, who are still in a self-centered, me-driven stage of your education (and life), may not be able to tell them apart. You might not be able to distinguish the excellent from the not so excellent, see which is which, or see who they really are.

Rather than denigrate anyone in particular or any universities by name, let me say that over the years, I have had the opportunity to meet many premedical students as medical-school applicants whom I was interviewing. They have come from many different universities. There have also been many premedical students who have found their way to my office in a roundabout way. The majority of the latter have come for a little extra advice and counseling.

Sadly, and very surprisingly, there have been quite a few who have had no clue as to what it takes to get into medical school. In addition, they have had no clue as to how to position themselves in the most favorable, positive way to enhance their likelihood to gain acceptance into medical school. Over the years I have spoken with students who lacked the grades, MCAT scores, volunteerism, patient contact experience, leadership skills, research experience, or some combination of these deficiencies.

They should have had a premedical advisor who could have pointed them in the right direction. These students might have been helped if they had been properly guided and given useful advice. And just as importantly, they should have been given guidance in a timely fashion. What I mean by this is that they should have been meeting with their premed advisors on a regular basis and throughout their entire four years of college.

It is so important for medical-school applicants to be ahead of the game. Proper planning and preparation are critical. Every medical-school applicant should have his or her own individual game plan and strategy to implement his or her plan. It is not just a matter of getting the best grades possible and hoping to score high on the MCATs.

Careful and proper planning will enable you to schedule your courses in a way that will give you the ability to build on what you have already learned. Proper sequencing will also help you to maximize your knowledge and skill set when taking the MCATs.

Also, you should consider the efficient scheduling of lab courses and four-credit courses so that you do not overwhelm yourself with an impossible amount of work and poor time management. Efficient scheduling and time management will then give you sufficient time, accompanied by less stress, to participate in extracurricular activities, volunteerism, shadowing, and other application enhancers.

Premedical advising must begin early!

I also strongly contend that it should begin in high school, whenever possible. I do realize that there are many young men and women who do not decide to pursue a career in medicine and apply to medical school until they are in college.

It is already too late to first seek out your premed advisor when you are filling out your medical-school application. It is way too late to begin meeting with your premedical advisor when you have been invited to your first interview. If your application has deficiencies at this stage, it will not be a strong application. This is one of the major reasons for having a good advisor, and for you and your premed advisor to schedule regular meetings, and to initiate your meetings very early on.

If you have a choice or any say in who your premedical advisor is going to be, then by all means, take control and get the best advisor you possibly can. How can you do this? How do you go about picking a premedical advisor? It's simple. Ask.

You can start by asking your fellow premed students what they might have heard, and who they have found has been giving the most productive and successful advice. Then put in the request at your school. Each college has a different procedure. The correct and most appropriate procedure will be listed in your university student handbook. At some schools, an advisor is assigned to you, and you have no input. Being that the vast majority of premed advisors are excellent and will truly do their utmost to give you the best and most meaningful advice, there will be no problems. But in the rare case that you are assigned a less-than-excellent premed advisor, you are still not SOL. Review the guidelines in your student handbook and make the appropriate change, sooner rather than later.

Throughout this book I have been emphasizing that you must be proactive in determining your future. I have been guiding you and giving you constructive ways for you to take charge. You are being given new tools that you may never before have realized you had at your disposal. Remember: focus, visualization, good stress, and time management. And especially remember that you are going to create, write, direct, and star in your own movie.

Seek advice wherever you can and whenever you can. It doesn't mean that you have to take it, but be smart and always ask for it—and hear it out. Be smart in how you decipher advice. In the paraphrased words of Ross Perot, don't surround yourself with advisors who are going to tell you what you want to hear. Surround yourself with advisors who are going to tell you what you don't want to hear. Let me repeat that and boldface it.

Don't surround yourself with advisors who are going to tell you what you want to hear. Surround yourself with advisors who are going to tell you what you don't want to hear.

This is one of the most important messages that you can take home. Take it to the bank. Ross Perot said these words to me as I sat on a chair lift with him and skied with him in Colorado many years ago. These words have been among of the major tenets of my life and have served me very well over the years since meeting him. As I have, you will do well to take this advice from this man, one of America's greatest success stories. The author Ken Follett has written a terrific, exciting novel, *On Wings of Eagles*, based on the heroics of Ross Perot. No spoiler alert here. I strongly recommend that you read it, and I guarantee that you will be inspired.

I have had the pleasure of working with, and having my office physically located next door to, Dr. Ira Gelb. He is a retired cardiologist who practiced for decades at Mount Sinai Hospital in New York City and was assistant dean for preprofessional studies at our college. He created our college of medicine. He is a man who recognized a need in his adopted community. He is a man who didn't just look at his environment and let everyone tell him no. He is a man who had a dream and did not let the naysayers take his dream away. He had the insight and foresight to step out of the box and not ask "why?" like everyone else. Instead, he had the courage to ask "Why not?"

From the time that he first conceived and visualized his dream—from the time that he conceived, created, directed, and starred in his own movie—he never let anyone, anyone at all, take his dream away. Now his dream is there for everyone to see and for a community to be proud of. We have educated and trained hundreds of future doctors.

But Dr. Gelb did not stop there. He simultaneously created our university's preprofessional program. The program was molded so that preprofessional students were regularly exposed to the many facets of the lives of physicians and allied health professionals. The students are also given the opportunity to shadow many of the physicians in the community, covering the broad spectrum of the medical specialties. The program has been so successful and loved by students that all seats are filled within the first day of registration.

I guess you could call this program the New York City Marathon of programs at this university, based on its popularity. Hundreds and hundreds of students have gone through it. But that isn't the point. Dr. Gelb is the most amazing, passionate, and giving advisor whom I have ever had the privilege of knowing. Each semester, eighty-five extremely enthusiastic students take his class. Absenteeism is virtually nonexistent. Most of the students are juniors and seniors. And then Dr. Gelb meets regularly with each student. He tweaks their curricula, offers advice on better course selections, and helps them find further opportunities for shadowing. For the graduating students, he will pick up the phone and speak directly with his contacts at various medical schools with an enthusiastic personal touch. He always, and I mean always, has a smile and a word of encouragement. He does not tear down, and he does not instill false hope. A little nudge in the right direction can make a raindrop become an ocean.

It is important to have realistic expectations. A seventy-year-old man is not going to run 9.9 seconds for one hundred meters. Well, at least not in my lifetime. An advisor who is worth his or her salt will always encourage you and help you to help yourself in accomplishing greater achievements than you may have thought possible. Beware of the pessimistic or inept advisor who, through his or her ignorance, will hold you back or give you bad counsel.

Even if a student does not present with the strongest credentials, a good advisor will not destroy his or her dream. A good advisor might say, "Let's work together and see what we can do to make it happen." It's sort of a one-success-at-a-time approach.

My overworked, pessimistic, never-smiling premed advisor told me, throughout my undergraduate years, not to bother applying to medical school. He said that the competition was just too great, even though I had the grades. I am glad that I have always been a bit of a rebel. The more he said don't, the more I did. I wish I could say that his was an intentional method to make me work harder, but it wasn't. But every time he said don't bother, he increased my drive and strengthened my desire. I am thankful for that.

Getting back to Jacques Cousteau, I now can look back with the twenty-twenty clarity of hindsight. As I turned away, dejected, I looked back at him one last time. He was walking away. As he turned, he looked right at me over his shoulder, and with a smile, he winked.

I realize now the gift that he gave me so long ago.

13. The Narrative

The narrative is perhaps one of the easiest *and* hardest parts to complete in the entire medical-school application. It is, without question, one of the most important elements in the entire application process. The narrative is where you get to shine, extol, stand out, stand up, sit down (just kidding), show your stuff, and, best of all, define who you really are. It is in the narrative that you get to speak and emote freely. Even if you are shy, take heart. The narrative will help you to a great extent (more on this later, in the chapter titled "The Interview").

The narrative is where you get to write about anything. You can talk about your life, your hobbies, your dog, your grandmother, your proclivity for carving duck lures, or your trip to Outer Mongolia. By now you might be wondering, "What's up with this guy?" I have actually heard about every one of these topics, and there are some others that I can't put in print. Anyway, let down your guard, open a window, open the door, and take a step into your "uncomfortable zone."

We all have limits.

We all have created walls around ourselves, to some degree. It is just human nature for us to try to protect our inner selves and secrets by putting up some form of wall or armor. You might be thinking that you have a lot of those uncomfortable places. These are the places you are just not comfortable sharing with friends. These are the places you are absolutely not comfortable sharing with a stranger, particularly a stranger who has power over you.

Really, now, who wants to share feelings of anxiety, fear, and inadequacy or intimate and personal feelings with a stranger who is going to make a decision about you, based on what you say or write, that will determine your entire future?

Even though you are the cream of the crop—or, better yet, the cream of the cream—you don't want to appear arrogant or out of touch. If you display too much self-confidence, you will probably turn off whoever is reviewing your narrative.

On the other hand, you must not be too timid, either.

By now, your head must be spinning. "What am I supposed to do?" Why is it that just about all the other people you know who are applying to medical school seem to be more at ease and comfortable in expressing themselves, their wants, their needs, and their dreams? Why are you feeling like a basket case? Why are you the only one who has fear and the inability to put on paper the very intimate, personal feelings that will greatly enhance your ability to open the door and cross the threshold into medical school?

Let me tell you something that you may not expect to hear or read. Allow me to let you in on a little secret: No matter how you look at it, we are all the same. We all have the same basic fears and anxieties. We are all afraid of the dark. We are all afraid of fire. We are all afraid of the unknown. We are all afraid of public speaking—well, maybe not all of us on that one. You would think that our number-one fear would be death, but interestingly enough, multiple studies have clearly demonstrated that the vast majority of people in the United States list that their greatest fear is public speaking.

As a medical-school applicant, your greatest fear is rejection. But really, what is the basis of the medical-school applicant's fear of rejection? Is it based on rejection throughout life? That is doubtful. To have made it this far in life, and particularly in your education, you would have had to have multiple successes, at least academically. Small successes fostered further small successes and then even more successes until you realized that you truly were doctor material.

We all learn from trial and error. We have to take small steps before we can take big steps. We have all been there. Up until now, most of your academic achievement has been based on absorbing, assimilating, arranging, and then applying new facts and large tracts of knowledge. And then in a rather Pavlovian way, you have been rewarded with good grades.

As you apply to medical school and fill out your application(s), you are asked to shift gears and open up your mind and your soul to perfect strangers. It is these strangers who will evaluate you and your application—and then make a decision about your entire future. They will decide whether or not your dreams are going to come true.

Now it is time for you to open the door and take that next, seemingly impossible step to success. It is time for you to put onto paper—or should I say onto the computer document—your innermost thoughts and feelings. It is now time to let out the true feelings that you have held onto and have never fully expressed. You are now being asked to fully express yourself and your feelings to strangers—for that matter, to the entire world. This is one of the hardest steps to take in the process of becoming who you are truly meant to be.

Over the course of your medical lifetime, you will hear countless thousands of patients tell you their stories. They will share with you their innermost personal secrets. They will share with you their greatest fears and discuss with you their anxieties. Some will be straightforward. Some will be almost boastful. Some will be angry. And some will need you to pry out every detail that you may need to help them in their personal moments of need.

Before you begin to put your thoughts together, before you sit down and create, and before you start to write, this is what I would like you to do. Just sit in a quiet, comfortable place. Go to the place where you escape to—the place where you find solace when the pressures of the world really get into your head. If it is indoors, turn down the lights. If it is outdoors, arrive in the early morning or early evening— the time of day when the light is the softest. Now, just sit. Breathe in and out, slowly and deeply. Listen to your breath. Feel the flow of fresh oxygen as it courses through your body to your muscles, to your fingertips and toes, to your heart, and especially, to your brain. Let everything else go. Just feel the flow.

When you get there, you will know. When you have emptied your brain of conscious thought, you will be where you need to be. Then, as if by a miracle, it will come to you. The seed will be planted. Then, as you keep your mind in this peaceful place, the seed will begin to germinate and enter your conscious mind as a new idea. Now you are ready to begin your narrative.

Let the germinating seed of an idea grow. Feed it with your passion. Remind yourself who you really are, where you have been, and where you want to go. This is what the fertile soil of the subjective part of your brain will request of you in order to create and grow the thoughts and ideas that will determine your future.

This is a technique that will work for you whenever you have to sort things out or be creative. It just takes a little time and practice to develop it.

Now it is your turn to share and discuss and yet do it in a way that will get the message across most effectively. Let's return to the subject that I have gotten quite far away from. Let's talk about the narrative. There is an important principle that you must adhere to if you want to be able to write the most effective narrative possible. A little earlier I emphasized that in your narrative, you must fully express yourself and your feelings to strangers. I also strongly suggested that you don't want to appear arrogant or out of touch.

You have to get the message across most effectively. The way to do this is to construct your narrative from real life events and to be sure that it comes from the heart. *It has to come from the heart!* Let me say it again. *It has to come from the heart—your heart.*

For those of us who got into medicine for the right reasons, compassion is at the top of the list. In another chapter I have discussed compassion and what you might do in the world of volunteerism to feed and nourish your compassion. Your narrative is an opportunity, a wonderful platform for you to launch the theme of your compassion. It is in your narrative that you have an empty canvas upon which you have the unfettered ability to paint yourself as you truly are.

Your narrative should tell a story—your story. It is here where you can candidly speak about what makes you tick. You may want to write about what motivated you to become a doctor. You may refer to a single, epic event in your life that sealed your destiny. Maybe there was a series of events that synergistically propelled you forward into medicine. Perhaps you saw or overheard a tender conversation between a doctor and a patient. Or you were party to a conversation between a doctor and one of your beloved family members. Many successful applicants write about one or more personal experiences and how they affected them and made it abundantly clear to them that their only pathway would be in the world of medicine.

Another moving—and effective—subject is that of medical volunteerism in the United States or abroad. I can honestly say that every applicant and student I have ever met or spoken with who has done volunteerism abroad has related a singular event that was his or her personal moment of epiphany. Working with the poor, disadvantaged, and needy is a humbling and meaningful experience for every one of us.

I wholeheartedly encourage you to write your narrative first, before you fill in the numerous slots for all of your other multiple activities such as community service, volunteerism, outside activities, leadership, shadowing, employment, medical employment, clubs, and organizations. Once you set the tone for your narrative, it will set the tone for the rest of your experiences. These are the more abbreviated descriptions of your activities that you list and discuss in your application.

Jumping ahead a few weeks, or months, it will set the tone for your interview. Your interviewer will read and dissect (hopefully, to be fully prepared) your essays, and particularly your narrative. The interviewer's preparation will most definitely influence his or her opinion of you. Remember, you are going to emote and express feelings in your narrative.

You want your feelings to be fully felt and appreciated by the initial evaluator(s) of your application as well as by your interviewer. You want your dedication, focus, compassion, and passion to fully transcend time and space and to reach the heart and soul of whoever reads and evaluates you and your narrative. You want these feelings to carry over to and set the tone of your interview; and more than likely, they will set the tone of your final evaluation and committee vote.

I want it to be very clear to you—absolutely clear—that when you sit down and write your narrative, you should really take the time to express yourself and let it go. Let it go and step out of the safe little box of your comfort zone.

You must let go and soar into the realm of personal expression. Let it go and tell the world who you really are.
Now is the time to express your emotions and let 'em rip your heart open.

Remember: compassion.

Set the tone, and the rest will follow. Don't be surprised if it follows you and sticks with you from this point on, all the way through your medical career.

I am now going to present to you one of the many narratives I have enjoyed during the interview process. Names have been changed, and other identifiers have been redacted, of course. This applicant set the tone of her entire application, interview, and medical-school studies with this narrative. It totally influenced how I read, digested, and interpreted her entire application. It also set the tone of her interview—little did she know. I can assure you it was from her heart, just reaching out to express her "inner doctor." And yes, of course I have her permission to show the world what a doctor is made of. So sit back and enjoy. I did.

"We are going to have to open her up here in the office today," Dr. Smith told his nurse. I had been shadowing Dr. Smith for the past year when Dorothy came in. She had just had tumors removed from her ovaries, and once home from the hospital, he acquired a nasty bacterial infection. Dr. Smith put on his gloves and handed me a pair. "I get to help?" I thought excitedly to myself! He handed me the Betadine and showed me exactly where and how to sterilize her abdominal area. He injected a local anesthetic and began to reopen her newly stitched-up belly with a scalpel. He explained to me, as he proceeded, exactly what he was doing. He had to drain the wound before it got worse. As he finished, he reassured Dorothy she would feel much better now that he had drained her wound and started her on a new course of antibiotics. With tears in her eyes, Dorothy looked up, thanked us, and added that it had been "a long road to recovery." I didn't deserve a thank you, as I was just the student. I actually wanted to thank her, because in that moment, my drive to become a doctor became even stronger. In my two and a half years of volunteering at the emergency room and newborn nursery of Good Hope Hospital, I have learned more than I could have imagined. I have learned not only basic infant care and the principals behind triage in the ER, but I learned

many principles that cannot be taught in a classroom or learned from a textbook. I learned that good patient care and a friendly word to someone not feeling so great go farther than I ever imagined. Having a minor in Spanish helped me immensely at Good Hope Hospital due to the large Hispanic population. I was frequently asked to translate for the patients, doctors, and nurses. I especially remember Juan sheepishly asking me recently if I spoke Spanish. When I said "yes", I saw his face light up as I was helping with his new twin daughters. He was curious to know when the babies could come out from underneath the warmer because his wife was anxious to see them and was relieved to have found someone that could communicate with him. He thanked me as he hurried away to tell his wife the good news that she could see them soon. My experiences at Good Hope Hospital have taught me compassion, especially for those of other cultures, in addition to instilling in me a deeper passion for a career in medicine. In addition to volunteering at the hospital, I began practicing the Korean martial art of Tae Kwon Do. The fundamentals are self-control, courtesy, integrity, perseverance, respect, and determination. A martial artist is taught to focus in the midst of chaos as well as being able to perform under pressure, which is also important as a physician. In my three years of practicing, I have learned how the skills that I have acquired will help me in my career as a medical student and future doctor. While pursuing my major in Biological Sciences, I worked at The Grand Hotel Resort. In my almost six years at the hotel, I have been taught to uphold the standards of a five-diamond resort, which is the highest ranking a resort can have. Not only has my job allowed me to pay for my college education, but it has taught me how to work and compromise with a diverse clientele. I also spent time conducting research with Dr. John Smith. The findings of our research have been published in the Journal of Scientific Discovery. I look forward to using my range of experiences as a volunteer, researcher, and foreign language speaker in my future career as a physician. The patience and understanding that I learned through working with various cultures at the resort will be invaluable as well. In my years as a medical student and on my road to becoming the doctor I have always dreamed of becoming, I expect to use the discipline, courtesy, integrity, and determination that I have learned from practicing Tae Kwon Do.

The key is to inject your heart into what you are writing. Pull from deep within your soul the very thoughts and sentiments that have brought you to this exact point in your life. You are now standing at the threshold to your future.

Let it rip. Let go. Now is the time to express yourself in the most candid, honest, and meaningful way that you are capable of. It is time to pull from within and create a narrative that will grab the attention of any and all who read it.

When I say grab their attention, I mean in the heart-grabber department. Let them feel your triumphs as well as your defeats. Open up the floodgates of compassion and passion. Make 'em cry. Now is not the time to be shy. But don't brag and don't let that ego of yours get in the way (more on this shortly).

Bring in your own experiences, especially the health-care-related ones. Maybe you took care of your grandmother, an aunt, or a friend. You can speak of your experiences overseas while volunteering to help indigenous peoples all over the world. How about the time when you were working at a soup kitchen and applied a makeshift bandage to an old man's hand, and then he looked up at you with his clouded, rheumy eyes to say thank you? That was the moment when you felt it. That was the moment when you were hooked.

That was the moment when you really knew that you had no other choice in life but to be a doctor. That was the moment that changed your entire life. Your destiny reared up right in front of you and pushed you onto a very special road: a life of ministering to the sick and needy.

That is what you should be writing about and including in your narrative.

We all have opportunities every day when we can make a choice—a choice of service to ourselves or to give of ourselves in serve to others.

This is the stuff of narratives. So dig deep into your memory and pull up the events that have made a huge difference to you. And better yet, pull up the events that have made a huge difference to you while you were making a huge difference to and for others, especially in their moments of greatest need.

Having just shown you an example of a beautifully written narrative, let me show you an example of what you may not want to write.

I live and breathe Martial Arts. Ever since I was a young boy, I have dreamed of becoming the next Bruce Lee who is probably the greatest martial artist of modern times. Watching him fight and seeing how he is able to get his way, inspired me to follow in his footsteps. I began my training when I was in middle school. Three days each week my parents would drag me to the studio to train. From an early age I have demonstrated my dedication to achieve and be the best. Then, through high school and college, I had to work really hard to find the time to squeeze my studies in. Even though I was able to get really good grades, I continued to improve my martial arts skills. In fact, I entered quite a few competitions and actually won quite a few. I was given the opportunity to intensively study martial arts in Japan for a year. While I was there I shadowed a doctor, once a month, at his private clinic. The experience was very exciting. He really inspired me. I also entered a few local competitions and did really well. So here I am now, on the brink of entering medical school. I am very excited and can't wait to start helping people. In fact I plan to incorporate my martial arts training. After all, the martial arts are like medicine in that hard training, dedication, and putting the time in will get you what you want. I also plan on training every day so that I can keep up with my martial arts skills.

I don't think that I need to explain to you the problems with this narrative. I actually read one just like this a few years ago. Needless to say, this applicant was not accepted to medical school.

Your narrative does not have to be medical. It does not have to be about volunteerism. It doesn't even have to be particularly sentimental. The idea is to portray yourself in such a way as to most effectively, and humbly if possible, demonstrate the personal qualities that you possess.

Narratives can take many different forms. The point is that you are being given an amazing opportunity to really present yourself in the best way possible. It is your opportunity to be the best advocate for your admission to medical school

As I have already indicated, you have to really work hard at it to be able to present just the right amount of humility by throwing out your ego while at the same time demonstrating the strong, wonderful qualities that you possess. You must effectively demonstrate the very qualities that medical schools are looking for to help them choose you, a most desirable applicant, to fill one of the few coveted spots that they are offering.

This is the time for you to highlight your compassion and passion, as well as your volunteerism. It is imperative that you incorporate these important qualities into your narrative.

Do not overdo it. Do not be melodramatic.

It is important to have someone else review all of the essays in your application. It would be wise if you did not ask your parents, grandparents, or significant other to do the review. The best-case scenario would be to ask a disinterested, honest, and educated person who, ideally, will read and give you honest and constructive feedback. Your parents and grandparents, and significant other will not be objective. They will tell you what you want to hear.

Remember: "Surround yourself with advisors who will tell you what you don't want to hear."

Write about an interesting experience through which you can show where you made a difference and how the experience affected you.

You may want to write about an episode (or episodes) where you made a difference, or one that caused a positive difference in you. You might choose to write about an event (or events) that taught you something new about health care, or lack of it, at some particular time or place.

You can relate an episode where you were directly or indirectly involved in changing or improving someone else's quality of life. How about a work experience in which you were faced with the need to make a critical decision that had far-reaching effects, or just a small effect, demonstrating your leadership skills?

Search your mind and dig deep. You have good stuff in there—everyone does. Ask your friends, family members, coworkers, teachers, and coaches about what they consider to be your strong points and best qualities. Don't be at all surprised if they come up with some excellent ideas about you that you might never have considered, or have forgotten, or, in your humility, were hesitant to include in your narrative.

Admissions-committee members will study your narrative. They will read every word you write, and they will do an extraordinary job of reading into what you write.

They will reflect and ruminate upon what you say. In fact, they will ponder and ruminate over what you *don't* say. Take your time while you put into writing what you really want and need to communicate.

Remember, you want your dedication, focus, compassion, and passion to fully transcend time and space and to reach the heart and soul of all who read your narrative.

14. LORs—Letters of Recommendation

You would think that all letters of recommendation (LORs) would be terrific. After all, these are letters that medical-school applicants have directly requested from their professors, teachers, sponsors, preceptors, administrative contacts, and "influential" people. These are the people who are supposed to know the applicant very well and are supposed to be able to deliver a strong and excellent LOR on his or her behalf.

The LOR is a recommendation that medical-school applicants are supposed to ask of someone whom they admire and trust. Students should also trust the contacts to write excellent testimonials on their behalf.

This is a letter that you are asking someone to write for you. You can ask anybody whom you have ever met and had contact with.

Think about it—you can ask anybody! It is one of the few and far-between opportunities that you will ever have, in your undergraduate and medical-school experience, where you have absolute freedom and control of any particular circumstance. And this particular circumstance is a very large one. It's huge.

Your LORs can, and definitely will, affect your overall desirability as a medical-school applicant. You must really put time and effort into figuring out whom you will ask to write the hugely important letters that will attest to the high-quality work you do while also supporting you as the outstanding student you are. This must be a letter attributing qualities to you that will make you a definite first-round draft pick to the medical school(s) that you choose to apply to. Of course you will only ask for letters from professors, teachers, sponsors, preceptors, administrative contacts, and influential people who know you really well.

It all sounds so easy and reasonable. Unfortunately, it doesn't always work out that way.

I am sorry to tell you that it is not uncommon for medical-school applicants to take for granted that if they request a LOR from someone, it will be just that—a "recommendation."

Let's just stop and think about that for a moment. Most students request LORs from the professors of the biggest and most popular classes. Unfortunately, these are often the same professors who have a very busy teaching load and, in addition, a resultant administrative obligation to these classes. Add to that the extra administrative obligations to their respective departments.

More than likely, you are not the only one requesting LORs from these professors. It could be that twenty other students have beaten you to the punch. If that is the case (and it probably is), then it would be a setup for a boring, lifeless, and uninformative carbon copy of a letter—a letter that will look like the snowstorm of letters that medical-school admissions committees have to sift through and ponderously labor over.

Typically, a LOR will have an introductory paragraph naming the student applicant. This will be followed by a brief attestation to the character and attendance of the student in that professor's class. This will be followed by a boring liturgy of the details of the class and/or research that the letter writer is involved in. I am talking really boring—boring to the point of putting the medical-school admissions reviewer to sleep. Then the reviewer will lose enough focus from the fatigue of boredom that he or she will not be able to effectively complete the remaining review of your application.

This is followed by a couple of paragraphs attesting to how well you have numerically done on exams. Your overall ranking in the professor's class is stated.

Finally, we come to the last sentence, which will say something like, "I recommend this student for admission to medical school." I have even seen, more than a few times, a sentence that says, "Even though I don't personally know so-and-so, I highly recommend so-and-so for admission to your medical school." How ridiculous is that? It can't get any more inappropriate. How can you endorse someone whom you don't know with a LOR to go to medical school and to become a future doctor?

Believe me, this kind of thing happens. You don't want it to happen to you!

A letter that is so bland and demonstrates so clearly that the professor or instructor doesn't have any sort of relevant personal knowledge about you will not help you in any way. Worse yet is a LOR in which the writer demonstrates that he or she doesn't even know you and has created the letter based on your assignments and exam grades. This kind of letter will, more than likely, not be perceived by the medical-school admissions committee as neutral but will actually hurt your application and admission prospects.

If you are going to request a LOR from a professor who teaches a large class, there are a few steps that you can take that will absolutely enhance your professor's opinion of you and will help him or her personalize your letter.

The first step, of course, is to do very well in the class and score high on your assignments and exams. You need to make it your business and a high priority to ask questions (intelligent, please) on a regular basis—one or two per class. Your questions need to demonstrate that you have absorbed the new information from the current lecture and are seeking to, or are able to, apply this new knowledge in a defined application or in an abstract, useful way.

An example would be that in an undergraduate human physiology lecture, you have learned that a low level of potassium (hypokalemia) in the blood can lead to disturbances in the normal rhythm of the heart. You remember, from a previous lecture, that severe diarrhea can result in low potassium levels in the blood. You then might raise your hand and ask, "If someone has severe diarrhea, can that lead to an abnormal rhythm of the heart?" Well done! Your professor will remember these insightful moments and comment on them in your LOR.

Another reward of studying diligently and being well prepared for your class is that it will enable you to answer the questions that your professor directs to your class during lectures. Trust me, the students who answer the big questions are the students who stand out. Your professor will remember these insightful moments, too, and comment on them in your LOR.

From time to time, you should meet with your professor immediately after a lecture, while he or she is still in the lecture hall or classroom. Ask an intelligent question or offer an insightful comment or observation directly pertaining to the lecture material. This is another way to help your professor remember you and reinforce his or her opinion of your excellent participation in class.

It is very important that you make a point to schedule periodic meetings with your professor at his or her office during office hours. This will help you establish a good rapport and add more personalization to your relationship (professional!) with your professor.

The point is that you want to establish a relationship and be well-known to your professor—or anyone who is going to write a LOR for you. Those who write your LORs need to know your strengths and be familiar with your coursework and grades. They need to be familiar with your insightful classroom contributions and how you are an expert at clarifying difficult points of information. They need to have witnessed how you are able to interpret and apply new knowledge.

You really have to know whom you are asking to write a letter for you and have a thorough understanding of what they know about you— and what their opinion is of you. You must have a handle on how you are doing in that class and have a good idea of your class ranking.

You had better be absolutely sure about how your letter writer feels about you.

Most professors and instructors will be frank with you as to how well they know you and the level of comfort they have, or *do not have*, in writing a LOR for you.

I have had students I didn't know ask me to write LORs for them. I am not talking about my medical-school students or my graduate students. I am referring to premedical students who might have heard me give a lecture or heard my presentation as a participant on a panel at a meeting. I always reply frankly, and quickly, that I do not know them well enough (not to be insulting by saying "not at all") to write them a LOR. It gets a lot dicier when a student asks me to write a letter, and as hard as I may try, I can't find a positive or even neutral thing to write about him or her.

To avoid hurting a student's chances of being accepted to medical school because of a negative or, as previously discussed, boring letter, I have politely indicated that I don't really know the student well enough to write a LOR. When a student becomes a little too persistent, I frankly tell him or her that I cannot in good conscience write a positive letter. So far, that has put an end to those rare, not well-thought-out types of requests.

As a long-term reviewer of medical-school applications, as well as having interviewed many medical-school applicants over the years, I have actually seen letters that have had the wrong name or multiple names inserted in a few different locations within the body of the letter. Obviously these were cut-and-paste form letters. How embarrassing that was for all parties involved.

Here is where things can get interesting—unfortunately interesting. There are some professors and instructors who will be asked to write a LOR for a student whom they don't really like or about whom they don't have anything positive to say. They will go ahead and write the letter anyway, and they will write it with either a totally flat affect or actually include negative comments.

This is the *kiss of death.*

To make matters worse, they might even state (and I have seen it), "Do not take [admit] this student."

With this kind of statement in a supposed LOR, you can kiss medical school good-bye. In addition to the direct negative impact of such a letter, it also clearly demonstrates to medical-school admissions committees that you have poor judgment.

You should consider taking some classes that are small in size, with perhaps ten to fifteen students. An upper-level course would be even better. If you want to score a slam dunk and kill two birds with one stone, make sure that it is an upper-level science course. The second bird is the ability to demonstrate your capability and capacity to excel in a more demanding and intensive science class. What about the first bird?

The first bird—and I won't use this metaphor anymore—will be for you to develop a meaningful, significant relationship with your future letter writer.

No, I don't mean go out on a date with your professor—very bad idea—but do develop a meaningful *professional* relationship.

A smaller class will allow you to stand out and shine, without being the "gunner student" that you might have to be in a large-size class.

Your ability to lead discussions, work well with your classmates, display enthusiasm, and exhibit mastery of the subject matter is greatly facilitated in the smaller-class setting. You will definitely be noticed, and your direct impact in class will help your professor to write a positive, meaningful LOR for you.

Don't just stop there. You will now have the perfect opportunity to spend a few minutes each day, after class, to ask questions and to *subtly* demonstrate your understanding and mastery of the subject. Your more personal professional relationship with your professor and the positive attributes that you have constantly displayed will result in the very best type of letter that you can possibly obtain.

At some universities, rather than have their premedical undergraduate students forward each of their LORs directly to AMCAS to be individually added to their medical-school application, there is a policy for each medical-school applicant coming from that particular university to forward his or her LORs to that particular university's premedical/preprofessional committee. This committee will then formulate a single LOR that will include quoted excerpts from the separate LORs. They will paint an overall picture of the applicant and support each attribute and quality with these excerpts.

The premedical/preprofessional-committee letter will thus be organized, literate, and as supportive as possible. The premedical/preprofessional-committee letter simplifies the review process by medical-school admissions committees and minimizes reader fatigue. This letter is usually constructed and written in a better style than individual LORs.

The downside is that these letters tend to eliminate much of the personal touch and feeling that individual LORs can so effectively transmit.

Another downside is that premedical/preprofessional LORs will try to objectify you, the applicant. They include class rankings based on your overall GPA. This is usually objective and can be good if you are in the top 10 percent of the class or better. However, individual LORs will leave out class-standing percentage rankings if you are not top tier.

An additional downside of the premedical/preprofessional letter is that arbitrary word rankings are not consistent among those universities that use word rankings. This inconsistency can lead to confusion. Each university has its own arbitrary verbal ranking system. They use terms such as "outstanding," "excellent," "superlative," "good," and "average." What might be considered superb at one university may be considered merely good at another. They will define what each of these words translates to, in ranking, within the introduction to the compiled LOR.

Once completed, the singular letter composed by the premedical/preprofessional committee is forwarded to AMCAS and then, within the body of the AMCAS application, to the medical schools to which you are applying.

The premedical/preprofessional committee's LOR can work in your favor or detriment in another way.

The goal of the committee is to get you into medical school. Committee members will do all that they can do to enhance the reputation of their respective university premedical programs. A higher number of admissions into medical school equates to a finer reputation for the individual universities. As a result, when committee letters are reviewed by medical-school admissions committees, it is well understood by all that the praises heaped upon the medical-school applicant may very well be inflated, biased, and self-serving of the university, and therefore they may not be viewed as favorably as individual letters.

Another possible disadvantage is that you have a single letter, not three or four. If the premedical/preprofessional-committee letter is flat or bland, it will work against you. Even worse is the rare case when the committee letter contains one or more negative comments about you. In the scenario of three or four individual letters, not a committee letter, if you get one bad letter, the other letters might balance any less-than-favorable comments with stronger statements and comments than are contained in the one bad letter.

You must be careful and selective regarding whom you ask to write your LORs for individual personal letters or letters submitted to a premedical/preprofessional committee for a compilation letter.

When submitting individual LORs, I strongly urge you to submit only the number of letters that you are asked to submit and *no more*. Letters that are submitted in numbers more than the usual three or four that are requested can become burdensome for the reader. It can become an ordeal for many admissions-committee reviewers to read five or six letters, and they will shut down.

Take a moment and think about some of the burdensome reading assignments you have had over the years while you have been working on obtaining your degree. If you had three assignments that pretty much delivered the same message, but by three different authors and experts, you were able to work your way through them. Now, think about having to read seven or eight assignments that all say pretty much the same thing. I think you get the picture.

Here is an important LOR tip: *do not ask an elected official or an elected member of government to write a LOR for you!*

First of all, these letters are commonly bought with big campaign donations by parents and therefore reflect extremely poorly on you. You are also putting the individual politician on the spot. The person doesn't want to lose your vote, your parents' votes, or your grandparents' votes, and neither does he or she want to lose a potential donation in the future.

I can honestly tell you that these letters are horrible and will only hurt your application. They are usually pretty cheesy, and it is quite obvious that the writer, in almost all cases, does not know much about you or, for that matter, anything at all about you.

As with most clear, direct warnings, there is an exception. If you truly know the politician or official well, and he or she really knows you well, then by all means, ask that person for a LOR. You must be certain that the person can write a LOR for you that will reflect the same depth of knowledge of you, your work, your character, your intelligence, your success, and your compassion as would appear in a letter written by a professor or instructor who knows you very well.

The only thing less meaningful than a LOR from a politician is a letter from a personal friend. Unless there is something in a friend's letter that is so spectacular that it will send you into the stratosphere and move you directly to the front of the line, don't even consider it. Just don't ask a personal friend to write a LOR for you.

An example of the type of personal letter that will possibly help you is one that is written by a personal family doctor or religious leader who knows you exceptionally well and can recount a lifetime of great deeds on your part. For most of us, that is not likely to happen. So stay away from the personal letters.

If you have spent a great deal of time doing volunteer work, and I mean quality volunteer work, then you might want to request a letter from a senior member of the facility, volunteer team, or, if possible, a volunteer physician whom you have worked with during the experience. This is an excellent opportunity for someone who has truly witnessed your efforts and observed your true nature to write a letter that will be able to extol your outstanding qualities under more difficult and meaningful circumstances.

Or, as an alternative, spending a prolonged period of quality time with one physician—in his, or her, office, making hospital rounds, visiting the emergency department, or even going to the operating room—will enable him or her to observe you and write a truly first-hand account of his or her experience with you.

More so than with any letter from a classroom, a letter from a physician who has worked with you "in the field" will provide an opportunity for the letter writer to portray your qualities of passion and compassion. It will speak volumes to any reader and testify to your future as a caring, giving doctor. This type of letter speaks directly to any medical-school admissions committee-reviewer.

The LOR is just part of the equation that determines whether or not you receive an invitation for an interview to any given medical school. Of course, different medical schools will have different criteria as to how they do this.

Keep in mind that your LORs to any given medical school will more than likely be read by a few reviewers. The first review will be by the primary application reviewer, who will get a sense of who you are and then score your entire application. Then, if and when you are invited for an interview, your letters will be read again by your interviewer or interviewers. The letters will be read with the full understanding that the interviewers will be meeting with you the next morning or in the next few days.

What they read will linger in their minds and will most definitely influence how they perceive you. So do yourself a huge, important service: think long and hard about whom you ask, or don't ask, to write a LOR for your medical-school application.

15. Ace Up Your Sleeve

This is perhaps one of the most interesting and controversial subjects that I am going to discuss with you. It is a subject that most medical-school admissions committees either embrace or struggle with.

I am going to propose to you—no, better yet, I am going to demonstrate to you and convince you—that the "ace up the sleeve" is one of the most useful and intriguing strategies that you will be able to utilize to your complete and total advantage throughout the entire admissions process—*if, and only if, it is apropos to your particular situation.*

In the not-too-distant past, the makeup of almost every typical medical-school class in the United States was homogenous. If you look at almost every photograph, of almost every medical-school graduating class, in the United States during this prior time, you cannot miss the fact that you see an obvious predominance of Caucasian men. There were very few exceptions, most notably Howard University College of Medicine in Washington, DC, and Meharry College of Medicine in Nashville, Tennessee. Both schools were founded in the latter part of the nineteenth century.

With the great upheavals of social consciousness that began during the 1960s and continued on well into the 1970s and 1980s, the picture of the student body of medical schools began to shift. The civil rights movement began to crack into, and then burst apart, one of the last bastions of the "exclusive men's club" that pervaded the medical-school culture and medical profession in general.

During the civil rights movement, brave men and women, including Rosa Parks, Dr. Martin Luther King Jr., James Meredith, and many others, paved the way for any and all Americans to be treated equally when enrolling into schools of higher education, including schools of medicine.

The women's movement also grew and had a significant impact during this period. Prior to the 1970s, a typical medical-school class of one hundred to two hundred students may have had one or two women in it. This was another example of the exclusive men's club that prevailed in the culture of medicine. The men's clubs of medicine were torn apart as a result of the dedication, sacrifices, and hard work of Gloria Steinem, Shirley Chisholm, Bella Abzug, Betty Friedan, and countless others.

The eleventh oldest medical school in the United States is the George Washington University School of Medicine. It was founded in 1824. One year shy of its 150th anniversary, the college of medicine opened the then-new state-of-the-art facility in the fall of 1973. The freshman class of 150 students had finally altered the landscape of the medical-school student body—dramatically! Almost 50 percent of the class were women. Unheard of! Unbelievable!

Lecture material and presentations had to be revised to be social and politically correct, and in a hurry. Whew, fun times. Many of the professors made politically incorrect and inappropriate comments. Slide presentations (PowerPoint was developed decades later) that had not been updated in years were often "booed" at by the student body—males and females.

Yet, as hard it is to believe today, when this class graduated in 1978, many specialty selections were limited to men only, or only a few spaces were grudgingly awarded to graduating female medical students.

Now, decades later, almost no one gives gender a second thought. As I look at current medical-school classes, I don't see gender bias. Women applying to internships and residencies are free to pick and to be chosen on their merits. Women are no longer relegated to the "soft residencies."

In fact, when I have discussions with current-day medical students and medical-school applicants, male or female, regarding this particular issue, the vast majority are not even aware of the blatant gender bias that existed up until just one generation ago. Wow, as the old Virginia Slims television commercial used to say (you might want to Google it), "You've come a long way, baby." The very essence of this commercial was sexist. However, in the context of our discussion, it is most appropriate.

Today, being female is not a plus or a minus in the application process to the vast majority of medical schools. Being female or male is just a statement of fact, as it should be.

Numerous studies regarding career choices and future demographic decisions of medical students demonstrate that many medical students apply for residencies that are within the same state and geographic region of their medical school.

There is also a strong number of graduates of residency programs who tend to stay and set up their private practices or group practices in communities in reasonable proximity to where they did their residency training. Throughout the many years of residency training, residents in all specialties build a vast network of contacts, referrals, safe harbors, and potential patient bases.

So, when graduating residents leave the protective "womb" of their training programs to start their individual private or group practices, there naturally exists a greater comfort level in making the decision to stay local and utilize the network of contacts, referrals, safe harbors, and potential patient bases that they have worked on for so many years. Residents who stay local, or in reasonable proximity to their training programs, create a win-win situation for themselves, and they begin their medical careers with a running start.

It truly is a fast track to success.

Of course, medical-career success is also dependent upon the individual's knowledge, proficiency, skills, ethics, and medical professionalism.

This trend of medical students and residents staying local has not been missed by local, state, and federal governments. The vast majority of state-supported medical schools have been mandated to establish, or have independently established, policies that create a diverse student population that parallels the diversity of each state's population.

Another way to say this is that the schools have been told that they must create and maintain an ethnic and cultural diversity that reflects that of the states in which they are located.

The thinking behind the creation of such mandates involved the intention and hope of training and retaining future doctors to serve the vast cross section of diverse patient populations within the assorted geographic regions of each state. In addition, and ideally, the purpose of the mandates is to mirror the diversity of the medical graduates to the diversity of any one particular region.

Private schools do not receive the same funding as state schools, and therefore many are not as compulsive in their efforts to broaden the cultural and ethnic diversity in their student populations. As with private golf clubs, tennis clubs, social clubs, men's or women's clubs, and many sectors of our society, there is still a lot of room for improvement of social consciousness. Over the years I have watched with great interest the changing membership of Augusta National Golf Club.

I hope that by now, you might be beginning to see where I am going with this.

So what is this "ace up your sleeve" for which I have titled this chapter?

The US government and the colonial European governments have a pretty sordid, embarrassing, and unapologetic history of systematically destroying the original cultures of the Americas—North, Central, and South America. Many centuries have passed without apology. Yes, there have occasionally been minimal reparations. It has been only in the last few decades, rising out of the civil rights movement of the 1960s and 1970s, that there has even been any attempt to right past wrongs.

I will not dwell upon the pros or cons of the current staggering profits made in gaming casinos, and gambling in general, in casinos owned and run by Native Americans and often on tribal lands, or whether or not the few are flourishing at the expense of the vast majority. I will, however, bring to your attention that in the current medical-school application process, Native Americans have a golden opportunity.

So, now I know that you are clear with where I am going with this conversation.

Medical-school applicants of ethnic, cultural, or religious minority or from other diverse groups can now take advantage of years of injustice. At least now there is an attempt to establish equality within medical schools, medical graduate programs (residencies), and, as a result, within the general medical community.

If it is applicable and appropriate for you, now is the time for you to play the ace up your sleeve! Let's discuss it.

By now you have most likely noticed, or soon will discover, that on the AMCAS medical-school application form, there are two clearly delineated places to establish your ethnic, racial, cultural, and/or religious affiliation. This release of your ethnic, racial, cultural, and/or religious affiliation is a strictly voluntary disclosure.

When you fill in the summary and biographic sections of the AMCAS application with your ethnic, racial, cultural, and/or religious affiliation, this information will be noted upon receipt of your application at some medical schools. This information will also be seen by anyone who reviews your application.

You do not want to stop with just filling in the blanks. Remember, this is your golden opportunity—your ace up your sleeve.

You also have the ability to incorporate and emphasize, in your narrative and in the descriptions of your multiple activities information, information about your ethnic, racial, cultural, and/or religious affiliations.

For example, in the activities sections or in your narrative, you might state, "As an African American growing up..." Or you might say, "Working in a clinic in rural [Texas, Oklahoma, North Carolina], I was able to identify and commiserate with the patients because as a Native American..." Another thought could be, "When my parents and I first arrived here from our home in [Pakistan, Haiti, Egypt...], we did not speak a word of English."

You definitely want to work your "ace" into your application.

Do take advantage of this.

You are in a competition to get into medical school.

Once you are in medical school, you do not have to compete any longer. You just have to work hard, and study, and be adept at applying your knowledge.

In your narrative and activities descriptions, you might also consider reflecting upon the great hardship and difficulties that you were told about in stories by your parents or grandparents when you were a child. You might elaborate on these childhood memories and stories of how your family, and especially you, were molded and grew in directions and ways that no one could have possibly predicted or imagined, especially during those times of great trials and tribulations for your family. Who could have imagined then that you would be applying to medical school today?

This is the very stuff that has shaped and molded America into the great country that it is—that *we* are. We are the "Great Melting Pot."

Be absolutely sure, however, that you do not create a story that is too melodramatic. Tell your story and tell it in a way that truly will help the reader understand the dreams, hardships, successes, and failures of you and your family. Tell the story in a way that will grab the reader's heart and soul. But don't overdo it. Don't make it too operatic (overdramatized and sentimental) or extravagant. You are not writing a best-selling novel.

Your goal is to create empathy for you in the reader, so that you receive the special attention that you deserve.

Here is an interesting scenario. I even hesitate a little to bring it up.

This particular set of circumstances, although completely aboveboard, ethical, and legal, still vexes many medical-school admissions committees and is the cause of much debate. The coolest thing about it is that medical-school admissions committees can't fight it, or do anything about it. They must follow the rules.

I am referring to a very specific subset of applicants who come from various countries of the African continent. These applicants may be Caucasian, Semitic, or Asian. They are first-, second-, or third-generation Americans.

Here is the fun part. According to the rules, this special group of Caucasian, Semitic, and Asian medical-school applicants are totally African American—legally and by the book. These applicants are the real deal and therefore are allowed, and encouraged, to fill in the box designating them as African Americans.

For now, if you fall into this demographic, by all means, take advantage of it. Remember, as we talked about just a little while ago, state-supported medical schools, and many private medical schools, make it a priority to have their student populations reflect the population demographics of their state.

If you are African American, or, for that matter, if you are a minority student and not included in the above group, I encourage you to pursue your dreams with steadfast focus and certainty.

Although medical schools profess to not consider or use quota systems for the admissions process and populating future medical-school classes, many schools actually do so—but in an ethical and transparent way.

Many medical-school admissions committees have figured out how to give special and merited consideration to minority students. There is a place in the application to demonstrate hardship and adversity. Unfortunately, or fortunately, in the medical-school application process, this is the perfect time to turn your "lemons into lemonade."

Don't hesitate to do this, not even for a second.

When medical schools evaluate applicants, hardship and adversity are two heavily weighted parameters. Together, they are another ace—an ace that puts you into another pile (sorry, I still fondly remember the days, prior to electronic records, when applications were filed in individual manila folders, evaluated, and placed into piles) and will give your application a significant boost.

The ace of hardship and adversity is not necessarily tied or related to ethnic, cultural, or religious minorities. This category is based on the applicant's life struggle for survival. This category is reserved for those applicants who, against overwhelming odds and the numerous obstacles of a harsh life, have somehow managed to complete their undergraduate education and fulfill the requirements for admission to medical school. (See more on this in the chapter "Hardship and Adversity.")

There are numerous parameters and factors the medical-school admissions committees consider in making the decision of who (and who not) to admit to their next medical-school entering class. Many medical schools actually assign numerical values to each of the many parameters and criteria that are reviewed in making the overall decision, such as GPA, MCATs, LORs, research, community service, and volunteerism.

As you can readily see, any information and extra considerations that you can supply to the individual admissions committees of the medical schools that you are applying to will be of paramount importance.

When the admissions committee evaluates your application, you will want your "ace" face up on the table.

16. Hardship and Adversity

Many of us have lived, and are living, fulfilling and incredible lives that have inspired us and given us much cause to be full of awe and inspiration, as the wonders and mysteries of the universe, and even some of the secrets of life, have unfolded and revealed themselves to us. We feel this joy and harmony day after day, and almost every moment of our lives.

I truly hope that you have been able to join me in possessing this wonderful, positive outlook during your journey in life. Unfortunately, there are many among us who have lived life as a constant struggle for survival and a daily battle against overwhelming forces.

Of course, there are many who find themselves between these polar opposites.

Please allow me to clarify this last statement. Our fellow human beings who find themselves in the first and very fortunate group don't just get there by luck or by just showing up. They don't get there as a result of the alignment of the stars and planets. (Let's leave astrology out of this discussion.) They arrive at this positive and propitious state of existence and actuality by consistently being proactive and making things happen for themselves. They control their reactions to the forces of life and unhesitatingly self-direct forward, always forward.

Sometimes we can't control the outside forces that are thrown at us, either from time to time or on a daily basis. Sometimes life comes up with circumstances that are truly not within our direct control.

Sometimes life or circumstances will create a situation where good, ordinary people are put in bad situations—situations that they were born into or ended up in as a child, sibling, spouse, or just because.

In the words of George Carlin: "Stuff Happens!"

But, you can take heart! Admissions committees and AMCAS understand that there is a reality out there. They completely understand that it isn't always pretty out there and that life and circumstances can be harsh, even for good people.

With an unstable economy, many families have been faced with the unfortunate circumstance of the income provider(s), whether one or both parents, becoming another casualty of unemployment. Parental unemployment will then add a new and tremendous burden to an already working premedical student. Just being a premedical student is already very stressful. Add to that the necessity to work while taking a full course load. Now, add to that the recent unemployment of a parent or parents.

Prior to the parental layoff, the student held a steady job to pay for tuition, room, and board as well as all of the ancillaries. With the new set of circumstances, the premedical student is now faced with having to support his or her parents, too. This might make it necessary to hold two or more jobs.

I can't imagine how the student's grades could not be negatively impacted.

Extracurricular activities will be affected. Leadership roles will be affected. Volunteerism will be affected. Patient contact will be affected. Research will be affect.

Heck, why don't I just say it: *everything will be affected.*

What can he or she do? What is he or she *supposed* to do? What would you do if you were faced with this potential disaster?

Medical schools are fully aware that stuff happens—particularly this kind of stuff.

It's a funny thing, but I never realized before that "stuff" is a four-letter word.

As I was saying, medical schools realize that stuff like this happens (and not infrequently); so in their inestimable wisdom, the AMCAS has set aside an entire section on the application (in the primary application) for you to be able to claim hardship. They have also left a big box, right there, for you to explain, in detail, the circumstances of your hardship.

Do realize that any information that you place in the hardship section will appear on your application and can be read by anyone who reads your application. This information will be reviewed, and evaluated by, any and all medical schools to which you will be applying.

Tell it like it is and give the details, no holds barred. You need to explain the details and write with clarity. You also need to provide as much information as you can to make your case. Sometimes it will be quite cut-and-dried, and sometimes you will really have to go in depth to demonstrate how your particular set of circumstances is deserving of consideration as a hardship and diversity application.

This is another little ace up your sleeve. Play it wisely and place it on the table.

What you write about and how you actually shape your thoughts will add a lot of information about you and will provide crucial information reflecting your ability to face adversity and yet continue to focus—in this case, on your studies.

The information you provide will also highlight your ability to multitask under stressful circumstances. This is a quality that medical students and doctors must master to be successful. Did you consider that your statement of hardship might also give you the opportunity to highlight your uncanny, and still improving, time-management skills?

As you can see, being in a life circumstance that puts you in a disadvantaged position, or having a hardship that taxes you to the maximum, is actually a life opportunity, albeit not always a welcome opportunity. The trick, or better yet, the gift, is that you can meet it head on and accept the challenge. Then you can think of ways to spin it around and transform it while simultaneously transforming yourself into a stronger, wiser, and more experienced human being.

These are the opportunities that enable you to actuate the old expression about "turning lemons into lemonade."

There is a place on the primary AMCAS application within the biographic section where you can declare your disadvantaged status. In fact, this section is titled "Disadvantaged Information." When you click on the box and then "yes," a drop down will appear. It will be a new space in which you will have the opportunity to explain, in detail, the circumstances under which you have involuntarily, or even voluntarily, become included within the subset of disadvantaged medical-school applicants.

Once you fill in the Disadvantaged Information section, it will become a permanent part of your primary application. It is a factor that will be figured into and considered in your overall evaluation, especially for the reasons I have talked about above.

Remember, hardship and adversity are included within many medical-school application algorithms that assign a hard score to each medical-school application. The algorithms for these scores figure in GPA, MCAT score, leadership, volunteerism, research, extracurricular activities, and life experience.

The medical schools that use such algorithms are attempting to create a more scientific (objective) method and less emotional (subjective) method in the admissions process. At many medical schools these scores are utilized for determining the hierarchy of assignment and sequencing of medical-school interview schedules.

Hardship and adversity are heavily weighted when inserted into admissions algorithms at those medical schools that use them. At the medical schools that don't actually use mathematic formulas, hardship and adversity are still heavily weighted during the evaluation of each individual application.

We are all humans. Medical-school admissions committees do realize that if you come from a disadvantaged background, your grades will be affected because of your commitment to working and/or caring for others in your family (or extended family). They also take into consideration the fact that you will not have the extra time to be involved in research, community service and volunteerism, patient contact, or extracurricular on-campus or off-campus activities.

I strongly advise you to diligently seek to incorporate into your multitasking world a job that will provide you with more than one goal. First, this job must provide you with sufficient income. Now, imagine finding a job that will also give you much more than that. Imagine finding a job that will provide you with an additional benefit.

Make it your goal to find a job that will pay you sufficiently and will also provide you with quality experience. Find a job in which you will be able to gain medicine-related experience and that will also provide you with the ability to greatly enhance your medical-school application.

You might consider, for example, working as a nursing assistant. I discovered this option many years ago. As I worked my knuckles raw, I was able to observe and experience so many incredible events. As a nursing assistant, I was also exposed to the hierarchy that exists within any medical facility, be it private or public, large or small. This was a time that forged my attitude toward all allied health professionals and helped me understand what made them tick. It was an experience that I never forgot over all of the years, in all of my interactions with any and all medical personnel.

Another great job that will help pay the bills and open many doors to many medically related experiences is working as a hospital orderly. (Yes, I did this one, too.) The cool part of being a hospital orderly is that much of the job will expose you to various medical and surgical procedures. In fact, in many hospitals, the orderlies get to do some of the minor noninvasive and important bedside procedures, such as placement of Foley catheters in gender-appropriate patients.

Another benefit of being a worker in the health-care industry is that you will meet many of the doctors, nurses, and allied health professionals who will be your faculty and/or facilitators during the years of your medical-school education.

Remember, these positions are suggestions to help remedy your hardship status. Seek them out as paid positions.

Obviously, you will need to learn the skills needed for these specialized jobs. The training that you will need can be obtained on the job. Your supervisors and coworkers will be delighted to have you. They will also be amazed that, as a future doctor, you care to know about them and what they do.

This experience will make you a better doctor as well as a better human being. The knowledge, skill, and experience that you will acquire will be priceless. This will greatly enhance the section in your medical-school application regarding life experiences and medical experiences. You will also be able to demonstrate your devotion, commitment, and focus to your future life as a doctor of medicine in a humble, yet featured, understatement.

You have created for yourself a win-win-win situation! You have turned lemons into lemonade.

You will proactively ensure that medical-school admissions committees will be aware of your disadvantaged status and the adversity that you have faced. The members of these committees will very plainly see how you have overcome adversity and have clearly demonstrated that you are dedicated, focused, and compassionate—all qualities so desired in medical-school applicants and future doctors. Better yet, you will be able to demonstrate these qualities by "walking the walk" and not just by "talking the talk." Add to this the fact that you have done so in the face of the insurmountable obstacles that have come into your life. Wow!

You will be constructing quite an excellent case supporting your admission to medical school, right? When you write about your disadvantaged status on your application, you should write with passion. It is imperative that you write with the passion that we have discussed earlier. In doing so, it will come through loud and clear, and it will speak volumes in your favor and help define who you really are.

Most applicants to medical school have worked very hard academically to get where they are in life. They have learned a lot and have gained an enormous amount of knowledge. As a result, they unfortunately have been left behind in a major aspect of the maturation and growing-up process.

Many of your fellow medical-school applicants have been left behind compared to their friends and peers in other walks of life and career paths. Many have not gained an appropriate level of life experience or the social maturity that would be expected and appropriate for their age groups.

Please allow me to say kindly that they are delayed or have not quite blossomed. I say it in a way that a doting, favorite aunt might say it. They will remain delayed until they have faced some of the harsher realities of the real world that you, as an applicant with a history of hardship and adversity, have already faced.

Here you stand, applying to medical school, and you are already seasoned and mature. Here you are with life experiences and huge doses of reality that will enable you to settle right in.

And the great news is that admissions committees will already know this about you.
It's in your application!

From the life experiences you have had, they know that you have a great deal of the patience and the strength that are so necessary to not only survive in the world of medicine but to also embrace and thrive in the medical world.

One of the keys, or actually vital necessities, to being a successful medical student and doctor is creative time management.

Medical school places a heavy workload on your shoulders. It never lets up, not even for a minute, during the academic year. Thankfully, most medical schools will not schedule major examinations right after the students' winter or spring breaks. You will get a prolonged rest during these breaks. They are designed to be especially long so that you will be able to fully recharge your batteries and add more memory to your personal hard drive. During the rest of the year, and the rest of your life, you will be on a roller coaster ride that is called "life."

Don't forget to add to the formula marriage, kids, mortgage, social obligations, health and fitness, sickness (God forbid), and X and Y and Z. I think that you must get the picture.

Getting back to the point of this discussion, based on your experience and what you have written in your application in the section of "diversity Information," you have been able to clearly demonstrate that you have already come a long way toward becoming an expert of time management and multitasking.

Make sure that you get this message across clearly in your application and especially at your interview. Just don't overplay this hand.

Make your point, make it clear, and keep it humble.

State your hardship and adversity as if it was just a fact of life that you have had to face, that you have had to deal with, and that you have done so successfully.

17. Unconventional You

OK, you are an accountant, lawyer, engineer, financial planner, stockbroker, or CEO.

You can make it happen. You always manage to be a mover and a shaker. You are the go-to person. You always make it happen when nobody else can.

All right, all right, we have a whole lot of other people out there—the other "real" people.

OK, you are a lifeguard, bricklayer, tennis pro, lab tech, or stay-at-home mom.

It doesn't matter who you are, what you are, or how old you are. Well, yes, age can be a factor (more on this later).

We all have dreams.

We have had dreams ever since we were two years old. Don't you remember those first dreams? Don't you remember when you were asked for the very first time by your aunt, who gave you a cookie and pinched your cheek (real hard) and then asked the two-year-old you, "What do you want to be when you grow up?"

What was your answer? Did you say princess, fireman, astronaut, cowboy, or chef? Hmmm, where are you today?

I am willing to bet that an exceptionally few of you are doing what you dreamed of way back then. What are you doing today? Are you happy? Are you feeling fulfilled? Do you wake up each morning excited to go to work, to see what the day will bring you? Are Mondays just as exciting for you as your Fridays? They should be!

One of the greatest gifts you can have, besides your health and the health of your family, is to be able to look at life and think to yourself, "I've got it good," and to be able to truly appreciate what you have. This might mean many different things to many different people.

One of the greatest sources of satisfaction in life is to love your job to the point that it really doesn't feel like a job. *This is a major take-home message!*

Not everyone is a professional ski instructor at Vail, Colorado. Very few of us become mega-famous rock stars, go on tour around the world, and get paid bazillions of dollars to run around on stage. How many of us own a successful hotel on an island paradise in the Caribbean?

I guess you can see where my dreams might be. But I did dream, and I have achieved my dream job status, loving my job so much that Mondays equal Fridays, and every day is a holiday—and so can you!

To be happy and fulfilled, you need to think happy and fulfilled.

So, if you are an accountant, lawyer, engineer, stay-at-home mom or dad, school teacher, or CEO, you can always change your mind and get off of that boat—if you choose to. It is never too late!

Medical-school students who have changed their career tracks prior to applying to, and entering, medical school have a knack for doing well. They have portable experiential advantages that they bring with them to school—maturity, leadership, life experience, stability, worldliness, understanding of team dynamics, problem solving, and the list goes on and on.

I hope that you are taking note of these qualities and self-reflecting as to whether you possess some of them, so that you can include them and expound upon them in your medical-school application.

Many years ago while in the restroom at Washington's Reagan National Airport, I came to a startling realization.

First, let me explain. When I am traveling, a lot of the trip involves waiting (connections, flight time, delays, boarding), and my mind empties itself. This is especially true when being very tired is added in. It is during these exact periods of time that my mind becomes most empty. These are the moments of greatest opportunity—when the mind is simply blank (See the chapter titled "Certainty"). It is then when the simplest and most universal of concepts and thoughts pop into my head—and your head, if you just don't force it or consciously try to make it happen.

These are the kind of thoughts that—try as hard as you will—cannot be consciously conjured. They won't occur when you try too hard. But when you least expect it, with your brain empty, they will just pop up as clear as daylight.

So there I was, in the restroom standing (remember, I'm a guy) next to my colleague who was a very, very well-known, prominent surgeon. And as men are known to do, he began to brag about the numerous cases that he had scheduled for the next few days. On and on he went, reciting to me a litany of surgical cases that he had scheduled for the upcoming week.

At least, at first I thought he was bragging. Now comes the interesting part. It suddenly hit me like a sledgehammer that he wasn't bragging at all!

He was just relating, with total joy, what he would be doing over the next few days. He was just reviewing, much like a skier relating the runs that he or she was about to do or a golfer reviewing the holes that he or she was going to birdie and par in the next round of golf. My colleague was joyful.

For him, each day at work was like a vacation day. Wow, do you see it? How wonderful would that be for you? A vacation 24-7! Do you think that you might be happy with that? Enjoy a long and healthier life? Pay it forward to others? Well, I got it. And within a few weeks, I changed the entire profile of my private practice and, hence, my life. It was absolutely amazing. Each day was like a vacation day. Ski instructors, rock stars, and hoteliers had nothing on me.

Today, many years later, and after a few more personal metamorphoses, I still view each day as a vacation and a gift. In fact, Mondays are as wonderful as Fridays. When Sunday comes, I can't wait for Monday.

Is this something that you may want for yourself? Now, don't kid yourself. Really! I want you to reach inside and be honest with yourself. What is it that you really want to do?

Earlier in this book, I extensively reviewed with you what it takes to be a doctor. I discussed with you, in great detail, the attributes that make that decision and career path the most wonderful, rewarding natural decision. For those of you who are currently locked into the doldrums of "get up, eat, dress, go to work, come home, eat, get undressed, go to bed," this is the time to be honest with yourself and get off the conveyor belt.

It is never too late to change your career and life!

Take the time for the introspection that you have been avoiding. Take that inward look and ask yourself, "Am I happy with my career, my life?" I will assume that you have already come to the realization that you are not, and this is why you are reading this chapter, a chapter that is written just for you—the career changer.

If you are an undergraduate and have decided that your major in post-Byzantine lyrical syntax is not in your future, and you have had a calling to pursue a life in medicine, then you will not have a hard time of it. You might have missed out on a few of the medical-school course requirements that are usually taken in the first and second years of college, such as biology, chemistry, organic chemistry, and physics.

So, what to do? It's easy.

You can extend your years in college to five in order to fulfill these requirements. Another choice would be to scatter the course requirements over the remaining years of the traditional four-year degree program.

If both of these choices sound unappealing, there is another option. You can take these requirements in summer school. It is actually a smart, logical choice. First of all, you will be demonstrating your dedication, focus, and commitment. Second, you will not be as time-constrained and stressed as you would normally be during the school year, being that you will not have all of your other courses competing for your time. There will also be fewer students in your classes, which will allow you to have a much more rewarding and personal experience with your instructor or professor. And, more than likely, you will get the A's that you need to pull up your GPA.

Voilà! You have created the ultimate win-win strategy.

If you are a graduate student or have a graduate degree, recent or not, and have decided that being a computer analyst or commodities trader is not for you, then take heart; it is never too late. It might take a little more time for you to complete the medical-school application course requirements than it would an undergraduate, but you can do it.

For those of you who can't just drop out of life because you have a family to support or other financial and time obligations, you can still make the "big change" happen. The easier way is to continue doing what you are doing—let's say continuing your law practice—and pick up your prerequisites at night or, if you are lucky, over the weekend. Another option is that you can go to summer school to pick up the courses. And as I discussed previously in this chapter, summer school comes with its own inherent advantages.

Many medical schools look favorably upon older applicants—read thirties and forties. The applicants in this special group are almost always career changers. They bring something different to the table—maturity. Even in this day and age of "forty being the new thirty," medical schools have a lot to gain from these applicants. This special group of applicants is entering into medicine for all of the right reasons and brings with it a unique perspective to any medical-school class.

Many times I have observed how older medical students will very naturally buddy up with, help develop, and bring up younger, less mature medical students. I have also observed how often older medical students bring with them specific skill sets and a host of nonmedical knowledge that they are happy to share with their classmates.

Then, either by example or osmosis, the younger medical students seem to miraculously adopt this more mature way of thinking and approach to life. This more mature approach to problem solving and working with others almost automatically gets transferred and disseminated to many other fellow classmates.

I want to change the subject for a moment, and then I will lead right back to the wisdom and seasoning of the unconventional medical student.

Let me paint a little scenario for you. You have just finished your umpteenth premed prerequisite science quiz/test/final exam. It is just one more of a gazillion that you will have taken during your undergraduate years. You are working hard to achieve the highest GPA that you can possibly achieve. And so is everyone else in pre-med! You wait twenty-four to forty-eight hours to get your grade. Finally, it is posted on the wall in a desolate hallway, or in the class-room, or in an e-mail, or on Blackboard. When you receive your test results, you are alone, very alone. Your reaction is yours, very personally yours, to react in any manner that you see fit.

So what happens when you get a B+? Are you happy, satisfied, or fulfilled? Do you accept your 89 percent? Then you review the exam, and somewhere, deep in an essay, or right there in front of you in a multiple-choice question, you very clearly see an ambiguity or an alternative explanation of your answer. So what do you do? Smile, pat yourself on the back, give yourself a hug? Heck no! Like every other red-blooded, American-university-trained premedical student, you hightail it right down to your professor's office and have what we politely call a "discussion" regarding the "interpretation" of your response and ultimately your grade for this particular quiz/exam/final, which will then give you an A for this course.

Then you begin to "politely" discuss the interpretation of your overall grade for this course, which will ultimately affect your GPA, which will ultimately affect your chances of getting into medical school, which will ultimately have an effect on your career, your future, your life, your marriage prospects, or your ability to cop front-row seats at the next big concert.

Am I right? Did I get it all?

Thank God for career-changing, older, mature, unconventional students. They have gotten over this immature cycle of grade-inflating events a long time ago. What medical schools, and medical-school admissions committees, have realized is that these mature students are desirable for their personality characteristics, seasoning, balance, and the example they bring to a class of young, aggressive, hormone-laden medical students.

If you are a career-changing, mature medical-school applicant, take heart. Your application to medical school is very much sought after. But you still must have the grades, MCAT scores, and the other desirable attributes of a successful medical-school applicant such as those that I have discussed throughout this book.

18. The Interview

You may or may not realize it, but the interview for medical school is the *major wall* that stands between you and entrance into medical school. The interview is what stands between where you sit as the medical-school applicant and where you want to stand as the "accepted to medical school" future doctor.

The interview is where you have to get to. It is your goal.

The interview is where you need to focus your attention. The interview is where you need to shine and come across as the "must-have" applicant. The interview is where you can proactively take charge and be handed the key that will allow you to unlock and step through the door to medical school.

The secret to success at the interview is for you to be prepared—to the max. You should be able to handle whatever comes your way. Better yet, you *must* be able to handle whatever comes your way.

There is a *secret* to guarantee a successful medical-school interview. For that matter, there is a secret to succeed and blow them away at any interview. But we will come back to this point in a little while. First, some important background information.

Everything that you have done up until this point has, in essence, been in preparation to receive an invitation for an interview. Yes, you read that correctly. Everything that you have done so far—excellent grades, MCATs, service activities, patient contact experience, all of it—was essentially to get you to the interview.

It is at the interview that you are given the chance to make your final case. Just making it to the interview causes your chances of acceptance to medical school to increase exponentially. Across the nation your odds of acceptance will jump up to 30–50 percent. Yes, you read that correctly.

So, what do you think? Should you take the interview very, very seriously? My advice to you is to prepare for the interview as if you were studying for a final exam or preparing for your MCATs. The medical schools are holding out to you a key on a velvet cushion—the key to medical school. But you have to earn it over an hour or so—a very long hour, or very short hour—of an interview.

The first major "rule" for the interview is tell the truth, the whole truth, and nothing but the truth. Let me repeat that. Tell the truth, the whole truth, and nothing but the truth! Usually, if I want something to sink in, I repeat it three times. But I will spare you the third time. In my past life, whenever I discussed informed consent with my patients, I always explained everything personally, and I repeated everything three times.

Numerous studies have demonstrated that when presented with information, people retain approximately 50 percent of the information with the first presentation, 75 percent with the second presentation, and 95 percent with the third presentation. This really holds true. Try it with your studies or, for that matter, everything in life—you will see.

So remember, tell the truth, the whole truth, and nothing but the truth.

Ha, I just had to sneak the third time in there.

Sometimes, applicants will include something in their primary application that is an exaggeration of the truth, or worse, something totally made up. You would be surprised how, at the time of the interview, this "stretch" of the imagination or frank untruth just rises to the surface. If you put in your application that you speak Urdu, you had better be prepared for your interviewer to ask you something in Urdu. If you stated that you spent time with a medical mission in Kurdistan, then you had better be prepared to speak in depth about the people, food, housing, medical care, and general culture of Kurdistan.

One area in particular where applicants get caught up—and it can result in an unfavorable interview report—is research. If you include research in your application, the interviewer will expect that you really worked on a research project. But don't be too comfortable with leaving it at that.

The interviewer will expect an in-depth explanation of your research, your role, your contribution, and an explanation of what you might have personally gained from your research experience. So if you reported in your application that you were working on a research project that "measured the uptake of 6–3 alphaminodiphosphorointerviewase and a comparison of its immediate and long-term effects on tropical tree frog interstitial uptake of transadaptase," then you had better be totally familiar with and conversant on this topic. If your interviewers aren't already knowledgeable regarding this topic, by the time you are interviewed, they will be. They will Google it and learn it.

Don't be surprised if your interviewers ask some deep and specific questions about your research. They just want to be certain that you aren't full of "aerosol of bluff" (code for BS).

If you don't know your subject, it will hurt your interview evaluation. So don't report it unless it is real. Be brutally honest about your role on the project. If you were a bottle cleaner and reagent mixer, so be it. But be honest!

If the research is going to be published, or has been published, all the better. But do not list yourself as an author unless you really are going to be named as an author of the publication. It is just too easy for the interviewer to check this out.

If you are caught in a lie, your chances of getting into medical school are very much diminished—pretty much over. Lying would be a statement of your character or, more accurately, a statement of your lack of character.

Here is another subject that is very important—but thankfully, only to a small group of applicants. There is a space on the primary application in which you are requested to "come clean" about any university actions against you. This must be answered truthfully and completely. It doesn't matter if the final result of the action was a negative outcome and a ruling against you, or if the outcome was found in your favor and no further action was taken. If there has been a university action, *you must answer the question.*

Over the last few decades, most universities have adopted strict regulations regarding life and activities on campus for all enrolled students. Much of the focus is on alcohol consumption and drug use. All students are furnished with, or given computer access to, the rules of student behavior. It is each student's obligation to know and understand these rules. Violations are not ignored. Students who violate the rules and are caught doing so are confronted with a university action. Like it or not, the rules are the rules. There are also rules regarding fighting, sexual harassment, hate crimes, and indecent behavior.

Each school has a different policy for how any charges might be handled. But in all cases, students have the right, and are given the opportunity, to defend themselves. No matter what the finding is, whether guilty of charges or complete innocence, any and all charges must be listed and explained. The best thing that you can do in your explanation is to tell the facts as they occurred.

We all make mistakes in life. It is human nature to be forgiving. If you are remorseful and accept responsibility, and you can demonstrate what you have learned from the experience, there should not be any negative impact on your application.

If you are a repeat offender, don't expect sympathy or support from your interviewer. Most likely you will be asked why you haven't modified your behavior. Let me just say, repeat offenders considerably diminish their chances of getting into medical school. It also goes without saying that the seriousness of the deed for which an action has been filed will be another key factor for how you might be evaluated.

I have not designed this book to be technical but rather to help you develop the tools and skills that will help you get into medical school. For that matter, I have honestly designed this book to help you, the reader, to succeed in life; so, having said that, this next section is technical. Having just said the above, I will now completely confuse you by telling you that I will start the next series of thoughts with nontechnical stuff.

One of the hard, cold facts of life is this: "The first impression is the lasting impression." We as humans cannot help but judge each other. It is who we are. It is in our genetic makeup. Perhaps it was an errant mutation millions of years ago that increased the chances of survival of our ancient ancestors. I will even bet that Neanderthals didn't judge and Cro-Magnon did, and that is why Neanderthals became extinct. Heck, go find the movie *One Million Years B.C.* and tell me that those early Cro-Magnon men weren't judging Raquel Welch and giving her special treatment.

We as humans have been judging for a long time. Our whole legal system is based on judging. Innocent until proven guilty is a judgment. Guilty until proven innocent is a judgment. A host of information is obtained, reviewed, debated, and torn apart, but eventually, the outcome is determined by judgment.

When you go for your interview, you are going to be judged—period! You must make a great first impression, from the very first contact with the office administrator at the medical school with whom you will be scheduling your interview to the very last person who shows you the way out the door at the end.

I hope that by now you have learned when to turn on and turn off the street language. No "like this" and "like that." This drives all adults crazy. If you call anyone "dude" or "boss," just get up and leave; it's over. You will be judged negatively.

Make sure your hair is neat and your face is closely shaved (mainly guys). And while we are on the subject of face, I strongly, very strongly, urge you to remove any and all metal, except for conservative earrings. Despite your first amendment right of freedom of speech and expression, you are going to be judged by someone who more than likely does not visualize a doctor, or community leader, with random hardware displayed on the face or neck.

This discussion does carry over to tattoos, also. Tattoos have become popular in our culture for all sorts of reasons. Some like to demonstrate artistry, and others might be making a personal statement. The reasons don't matter. I am not judging. I am just recommending that you remove or cover any visible tattoos so that—even though it would be unfair—you don't make a bad first impression. I have had many medical students who have had extraordinary tattoos in all sorts of unusual and artful displays, but they were not visible at their interviews. Whether or not this is fair is not the discussion. The same goes for metal accessories.

Just be smart. You can give up some of your freedom of expression for a few hours.

Express yourself intelligently.

Although you might want to express yourself fully, although you might be used to expressing yourself through your body art, although you might not want anyone telling you how to look, this is not the time or place to draw your line in the sand. We live in an age of instant gratification and all sorts of public displays. This is an age in which so many people do not consider the long-term consequences of their actions, and how these actions might affect their friends, neighbors, relatives, or strangers, or themselves.

So many of us do not think about the consequences of our actions. What might seem like a small, inconsequential act might turn out to have huge consequences. Holding a door open for someone at the supermarket might have huge effects. Perhaps that one kind deed was enough to show someone that others care about him or her. Then that person goes home and doesn't take out their anger on his or her kids. And then the kids go to school and don't bully another kid. And then that kid sees that life might not be horrible. And then, and then, and then...I think you get the picture.

What are usually not so obvious are the results of our actions. Sometimes we see the cause (our action) and the immediate effect. But there are innumerable events that have occurred, and are occurring all of the time, that have far-reaching and tremendously consequential results. A child bullied today may, in a few years, become the guy at the mall who opens fire into a crowd with an assault rifle. Or a child complimented on her science project today may become the brilliant scientist who discovers the cure for cancer.

We live in an age where we are just beginning to see the primeval stirrings of a concern for our environment. Hopefully it is not too little, too late. We cast away our discards without a second thought or concern. Entire mountains of diaper landfills are created. Thousands of square miles of floating plastic and garbage perpetually sit in the doldrums of the mid-Atlantic. These are causes with effects that will haunt us for thousands of years—the time it takes for diapers and plastic to decompose.

OK, back to your interview. Your interview is an opportunity for you to consider your actions and their consequences. In this case, your actions have a short-term effect: being recommended for admission to medical school. And a long-term effect: becoming a doctor. This is not the time for you to draw your line in the sand of freedom of individual expression. You can do that later. This is the time for you to shine based on your strong scholastic record and outstanding personal qualities.

As we are discussing appearance, this would be a good time to take things a little further. I am sure that you have heard the expression "When in Rome, dress like the Romans do." I can't emphasize it enough: "When interviewing to become a doctor, dress like a doctor." It's actually pretty simple, as long as you remember that this is not the time to make a fashion statement. Remember, "When in Rome..."

The key is to look professional and to stand out, a little, in your professional display. You do want to make a statement with the way you dress for your interview. You want to state, "Here I am. Not only do I look like a professional—in this case, a doctor—I deserve to be a professional."

Don't push it too far. You should aim to look good, but not *too* good. You don't want the interviewers to resent you for any insecurities that they may have about their own appearance. But you do want them to look at you and, consciously or unconsciously, see the look of professionalism and dedication—the look of a doctor.

Like many applicants, you may look young, so it is doubly important that your clothing fit you correctly. If your clothes are too big or too small, it gives them the look of hand-me-downs from an older sibling and will put emphasis on how young you really are (or appear to be). This is usually subliminal, but as I discussed a little earlier, you are going to be judged, and the first impression is the lasting impression.

Now for some technical stuff. At your interview, wear a clean, unwrinkled, well-fitting dark suit that is appropriate for your gender. If you are a guy, wear a tie that is tied properly and snug. If you are a female and elect to wear a blouse, do yourself and everyone else a favor—wear an appropriate neckline. And for God's sake, do not wear sandals or, heaven forbid, flip-flops. And lastly, guys, do wear socks. Ladies, whether or not you wear stockings or leggings is a personal choice.

There are a few things that you can do right from the get-go, that can positively, or negatively, impact your interview. At some institutions you will be in a conference room with other applicants. Then you will be greeted by your interviewer, who will accompany you to a private office or interview room. At other institutions you may be the only one, and when you arrive, you may go directly to the interviewer's office.

Whether you are greeted by your interviewer in a group setting and brought to the interviewer's personal office, or you knock on the door and are invited to enter, there are a few things that you can do correctly, or incorrectly, to influence the interview—immediately.

Once you enter the interview room or office, wait until the interviewer sits down first or encourages you to sit down. He or she will indicate which seat is for you. I cannot emphasize this strongly enough.

Do not put any of your personal belongings on the interviewer's desk!

This is equivalent to entering a stranger's house and immediately making yourself comfortable in his or her favorite sofa chair. This is equivalent to trash-talking a complete stranger. It is a total no-no. A professor's desk is his or her inner sanctum, cave, and lair. You just don't want to enter a lion's den on unfriendly, aggressive terms. It is much wiser to simply ask where you may place your possessions.

More than likely, the interviewer, who has done this many times before, will tell you before you get a chance to ask.

Introduce yourself, sit down, smile (but not theatrically), stay silent, and wait. Let the interviewer initiate the interview.

I am now going to give you the *second* most important tip that I can give you for a successful interview. In fact, this advice will help you throughout your life when asked a question by anyone, at any time. OK, here goes.

When the interviewer asks you the first question, and all subsequent questions, *don't answer*. That's right, don't answer. Well, at least at first. When you are asked a question, sit still, look directly at the interviewer, don't speak, collect and organize your thoughts, and then answer in your normal conversational manner.

Make your point in a few simple sentences. Don't make it too short. *But please, don't make your answer too long*. Not only will the interviewer become distracted, but more than likely, you will also get distracted and start running off in another direction and lose track of what you really want to say.

Let's say that you are asked a question that you are totally prepared to answer. Remember, don't answer right away. Remain silent. Collect and organize your thoughts. Then look right at the interviewer and answer the question. Glorify in being prepared and bask in the light of self-satisfaction. But don't let it show in any way. Enjoy the moment. Remember, answer the question, and don't elaborate.

Now, for the *third* most important tip I will share with you: ***Once you have made the "sale," shut up!***

Don't say anything else until the next question. You can only ruin it. Really, it is very simple. I can't even begin to count the number of times applicants have been off to a running start and then blown it by running off at the mouth.

State what you have to state and then stop. Stop. Stop. Once you have made the sale, shut up!

Now I will reveal the most important and critical tip for your medical-school interview. In fact, this tip is essential for any interview, anywhere, anytime, for the rest of your life.

Almost everyone who goes for an interview has the same mentality. It doesn't matter what type of interview it is. It can be a job interview or perhaps an interview for the NFL draft. Maybe a law school interview. Almost everyone does it, and they do it wrong.

Almost everyone goes into an interview hoping beyond hope that they don't blow it and that they do get the job or position. This mentality already sets up an atmosphere of negativity and inferiority for the person being interviewed. Before the interview even gets started, applicants are setting themselves up. They are introducing doubt. They are introducing negativity.

You must enter the interview with a positive attitude.

Is that it? Is that the big number-one tip? In a word, nope.

The big tip is this: ***for every interview that you will ever have, from right now until forever, you are the one doing the interview.***

Easy, right? Well, actually it is. It will take a few major life interviews before you become an expert at this. But an expert you will become. The key is to have foremost on your mind the mentality of "I am here for this interview for you to show me, prove to me, why I should accept this position, why I want to come here." That's it.

It really is very simple. You must be in charge of your interview. You have so much to offer and are so right for the position, and you know it. It is their job to convince you that the position is right for you. In this case, the position is their medical school.

You will be floored by the results that you will achieve with this approach. When you step out of your current comfort zone and interview with this technique, you immediately (and subconsciously) increase your desirability and the interviewer's perception of you.

This works for all interviews. It boils down to wanting something for its perceived value.

As the Rolling Stones said, "You can't always get what you want." It is precisely the perception of something being difficult to obtain that makes it more desirable. In our culture we assign value to that which is difficult to obtain. By turning the interview around and making it clear that *you* are interviewing the medical school to see if it is what you want, you automatically increase your value, tremendously. You create and enhance your own demand.

You have the ability, the gift, to turn it all around. You have the ability to increase your desirability for admission to each medical school at which you have an interview. The key is not to overplay your cards. You don't want to sound cocky. You want to come off humble and desirable. You want to create an impression of humble confidence. You want to project your worth.

You want to subtly reverse the interview so that you are in the interviewer's seat. Hmm, not literally. That will get you in a lot of trouble. What I am saying is that you want to project the image that you are a desirable applicant whom the particular medical school really wants to admit.

The way you do this is to visualize, as you are being interviewed, that the roles are reversed. Really, visualize it with commitment, and it will become your reality. This is the major premise of the multiyear *New York Times* best-seller, *The Secret*, by Rhonda Byrne. If you put the energy out there, you can achieve almost anything—of course, within reason. You won't be flying above rooftops unless you devise a technique to grow functional wings.

I highly recommend *The Secret* to teach you how to develop and grow into this wonderfully powerful, positive frame of mind. It will change your life. I know—it totally changed mine.

There are different kinds of interviews, depending on the philosophy of the medical school where you are interviewing. The most common format is the one-on-one interview. This might be a single interview with one interviewer for one hour, or it may consist of two back-to-back half-hour interviews with two interviewers, one for each half-hour segment. In fact, the first interview may be the standard interview that I have been discussing above. (At the end of this chapter, I will supply you with a few of the types of questions that you might be asked).

If you have a split interview, back-to-back half hours, the second half-hour of the interview may be the same style as the first, but with a different interviewer. Or you may have the now-in-vogue "behavioral interview."

There have been numerous studies and presentations that demonstrate that the behavioral interview is a more consistent indicator of the qualities that predict greater success of the medical-school applicant as a medical student. The behavioral interview is centered on questions that are based on ethical, moral, and professional standards—all qualities that we wish to see in medical students and doctors. But really, why stop there? We should see these same qualities in lawyers, politicians (oops, that is a major oxymoron), teachers, corporate leaders, and so on. Hmm, I will have to write another book for them.

To tie this chapter together, I am listing some sample questions from the standard interview and the behavioral interview. Think long and hard about your responses. Don't memorize!

Memorized and canned responses are easy to see through. Practice asking and answering the questions to yourself, to the mirror, to your family, to your friends, and even to your dog. The more you work on your responses to each question, the more they become a part of you, your thinking, and your soul. As a result, you will be able to answer these questions at your interview without your responses sounding contrived or memorized.

SAMPLE STANDARD QUESTIONS

Why do you want to be a doctor?—This is the granddaddy of them all, and you will be asked this question at *every* interview and by *every* interviewer. I placed this question first to get it out of the way. Please review the chapter titled "Why a Doctor?"

What qualities should a doctor have when administering health care?

What leadership roles have you had?

What qualities should an effective leader have?

Who are your role models and why?

What role did you have in the research project that you have listed on your application?

Explain to me the subject and the results of your research.

What have you learned from the volunteerism (community service) that you have been involved in?

You have indicated that you speak a *foreign language*. Tell me of your future plans. Please give your answer while speaking in that language.

Why have you chosen our medical school?

What qualities do you have that are special and that will enhance the experience of your classmates?

What is there about you that I haven't asked and you feel that I should know?

SAMPLE BEHAVIORAL QUESTIONS

Tell me about a situation where, after you did something, you later found out that a policy existed that you should have followed. What did you do? What did you learn?

Have you ever been a witness to a classmate cheating? How did you respond to the situation, and what did you learn from the experience?

Tell me about how you handled a confidential issue in the past when you were requested to provide information.

Have you ever had a friend whom you felt needed help with a substance abuse or emotional problem? What did you do about it? What did you learn from that experience?

We all get overwhelmed from time to time. Tell me about the last time you became overwhelmed at school and how you handled the situation. What did you learn from the experience?

Do you believe that a physician should always be 100 percent honest with patients?

Then as a follow up...

What situations do you believe might allow for being less than 100 percent truthful?

Tell me about one of the greatest disappointments in your life, a time when you did not get something you really wanted. How did you respond to that disappointment at the time? How do you feel about it now?

How do you think your past experiences translate into success in medical school and the practice of medicine?

Tell me about a time when you had to "think outside of the box." How did it go, and what did you learn from that experience?

19. Conceive, Write, Direct, and Star in Your Own Movie

In this book I have revealed to you quite a few of the secrets of getting into medical school. You have read about some of the little things (and not-so-little things) that can enhance or detract from your medical-school application. I have discussed with you many of the factors that can make, or possibly break, your future in a career of medicine. I have provided you with various exercises to improve your focus. You have read how to capitalize on your ability to visualize. In addition, we have discussed how to enhance your absorption, synthesis, recall, and application of information. I have given you a blueprint on how to sharpen your study skills and levels of performance.

But, really, have all of these been secrets?

Perhaps it will be better if you view this book and all of the information that I am sharing with you as a bunch of suggestions, tips, and pearls from someone (me) with a little experience with the medical-school admissions process. But that wouldn't be accurate or reflective of why I wrote this book.

When you come right down to it, these chapters are full of all sorts of esoteric and seemingly unrelated tidbits of information. My guess is that while you have been reading these pages, you have asked yourself (quite a few times), "What is he saying? What is the point here?

What does this have to do with getting into medical school? What does this have to do with anything?"

After you have read it all, and not necessarily in any particular order, I have no doubt that you will see that you have been provided with a clear, concise, and well-thought-out strategy that will lead you to the doors of medical school. Also, in these pages you have been given the tactics that will enable you to address each of the individual aspects of the complete medical-school application (literally and figuratively) and will mold you into the complete medical-school applicant.

Whether or not you get accepted and pass through the doors into medical school is entirely up to you. It will all depend on your attitude, your openness to the suggestions presented to you in this book, and your willingness and focus on implementing these strategies and techniques. There is a lot of subtle information contained within these pages. Much of the information is straightforward and to the point. Reading those sections will be like reading a newspaper and seeing the information presented to you without puffing it up with editorial digressions.

Other extremely important information and life lessons that will absolutely augment your chances of getting accepted into medical school are contained within the stories and anecdotes that I have shared with you. They are revealed to you between the lines of the words that you have read in plain black and white.

Within the body of all of my lectures to my medical students, I illustrate the main points with this same style of stories and anecdotes. I always feel that I have succeeded with my teaching goals when I receive student evaluations of my lectures at the end of each course. Many of the students write that they are able to understand and retain the learning objectives of each lecture by associating the learning objectives with the stories I have linked to them.

The success of this technique of teaching is also verified by the e-mails I receive from previous students who are now in their residencies and private medical or surgical practices across the United States. I always get the warm feeling of a proud parent and can't help but smile when I receive these e-mails, because almost every one of them states that the anecdotes and tangents they listened to in my lectures have become triggers to areas deep in their memories that help them recognize, diagnose, and treat their patients in hospital wards, clinics, and private offices.

On first blush, you might have really wondered about all that you have read in this book. Let me assure you, if you have read everything carefully, understood it, taken it all to heart, and implemented my suggestions, you will accomplish what your intention was in the first place.

You will enhance the possibility and your probability of getting into medical school!

I have given you tools to understand and enhance your ability to focus. With the many references to focus that I have placed throughout this book, you are sure to see what a key element this is for your future life in medicine. Focus is what sets the professionals above the amateurs. Focus is what enables you to multitask, yet pay complete attention to each of the tasks that you are involved in. Focus is what allows you to tune out everything around you and enables you to expertly address, and complete, the task at hand.

I remember the first time I saw Tiger Woods. He was a very young child on TV, demonstrating his golfing skills on *The Tonight Show*. Even then, I was able to observe his complete focus. If you watch him today during any golf match, you will see it in his eyes and in every fiber of his body—focus. In fact, from the time Tiger first picked up a golf club, his father, Earl Woods, who was also his coach and golf mentor, very cleverly conditioned him to focus. It was quite amazing and creative how he did it. Here is how it worked.

Each time that Tiger would set up his stance or begin his swing, his dad would cough, talk, produce noise, or make some distracting movement. Tiger learned to remain unfazed.

Tiger Woods is the epitome of focus.

You have learned about passion. You have learned that if you follow your passion(s), you will have an amazingly satisfying life. If you make your passion and your "job" the same thing, then is your job really a job? I think not. As I related to you earlier with the story about the airport in Washington, DC, my colleague was so passionate about his surgery practice that he could not wait to get back to his office and go back to work—his job, his passion. It is a wonderful, beautiful thing to wake up each day and pursue your passion. When you reach this point, you feel like every day is a holiday. Work is fun, your passion is being fulfilled, and life is wonderful. Really!

I totally appreciated and enjoyed my former life as a practicing surgeon. Now, as a medical-school teacher, writer, advisor, and motivational speaker, I find that my true inner passion is being completely fulfilled. Each day is a blessing and a gift. Every day I live my passions. Every day is a holiday.

More than likely, you would not be applying to medical school and agreeing to accept all of the responsibility that comes with it (why do you want to become a doctor?) if you didn't already have the compassion that the practice of medicine expects and demands. Giving of yourself so that you can help others must be done without hesitation or question. In fact, if you are truly compassionate, you do not view giving up anything of your own as giving it up. You don't view self-sacrifice as a sacrifice. A compassionate person or physician gives all of him- or herself without ever questioning or trying to justify it.

In fact, a great majority of medical-school application narrative essays display early childhood demonstrations of this beautiful quality of compassion as the chief guiding influence for the choice to apply to medical school and to become a doctor. In almost every application narrative essay, extraordinary compassion was displayed by a doctor, nurse, or physician's assistant to a beloved family member or to the applicant.

Compassion. It is such a beautiful, wonderful quality. It can drive the world, if only we let it.

When we discussed medical volunteerism, I emphasized an important caveat: you should do this over a prolonged time period. Many medical-school applicants demonstrate their volunteer time in a haphazard fashion. It almost appears as if they are seeking an Olympic gold medal for the quantity and variety of experiences. But I have asked myself when I reviewed these applications, "Where is the quality? What have they really contributed? What have they learned?"

It is not the quantity or variety of volunteer experiences that counts; it is the demonstration of altruism, commitment, and dedication that will bring notice to you.

And, of course, these are the very qualities that medical-school admissions committees want to see in every candidate they accept. These are characteristics that are intrinsic to the "great" doctors in each and every community. More than likely, these were the qualities that you consciously (or unconsciously) witnessed and that inspired you, years ago, to pursue a career in the practice of medicine.

You have worked hard to get accepted into medical school. You realized quite a while ago that you are very different from your friends, acquaintances, and classmates. You made a conscious decision to accept hardship and sacrifice so that you would be able to realize the dream that you are on the brink of achieving.

Remember, "Fifteen minutes of preparation will result in hours of surgery; hours of preparation will result in fifteen minutes of surgery." Proper preparation is the key to most successful endeavors. And yes, the ability to spontaneously think on your feet is also an important attribute and an exceptionally helpful tool to have along the road to achieving your goals.

All of the years of planning and preparation, the days and nights of sacrifice and hardship, have enabled you to get into medical school. Ultimately you are planning for the rest of your life—a life of being the best doctor you can possibly be.

You are now beginning to understand what an incredible gift you are being given—and have earned. It is a gift that so few people ever get to experience, even though it is a gift that comes with an incalculable responsibility. But what a wonderful responsibility.

You are being given the gift of healing. It is an awesome responsibility. To save life—a single life or thousands of lives—is the most awesome of responsibilities that we can accept. It is the highest and most incredible calling a human can aspire to. And just think about the countless generations of lives you will be able to ensure and preserve by saving just one life.

Never take this for granted. ***It is not a superpower, and you are not a superhero!***

You can be a hero—a wonderful, giving, dedicated hero who will make a difference in the lives of countless people today and tomorrow and who will impact generations to come.

This is your calling and what you have aspired to be. With this mission it is hard to remain humble and not let your ego take over. You must always be on guard to avoid this trap, because if you do let your ego get in the way, you will make poor decisions. Ego-driven decisions are almost always bad decisions. Ego-driven decisions are made to impress others and will cloud your thinking and judgment. When decisions are ego driven, they often will lead to errors of commission.

Errors of commission are the result of someone doing something unnecessary, inappropriate, or wrong. In the field of medicine, errors of commission are unacceptable and more often than not will result in medical errors that can seriously injure a patient, lead to an unsatisfactory outcome, or much worse.

This is different from errors of omission, which result from someone not doing something or failing to do something correctly. Although errors of omission can lead to medical errors, thankfully, in the world of medicine, these types of errors can usually be resolved. Errors of omission are based on timidity, lack of training, or lack of understanding. It takes a patient-supervising body to recognize these errors and provide the proper training.

As you can see, errors of omission are usually avoided with proper training and education. Errors of commission are ego driven and unpredictable, and they can be disastrous. At this stage you are most likely in the most humble, and humbling, part of your life. Avoid the ego trip, and you will almost certainly be able to give your patients and community that which you so easily and naturally give today.

Your attitude toward your future patients, and colleagues, is really the bottom line. How you perceive and react to your fellow human beings is your signature in your community. It is also your attitude that determines how you are perceived and reacted to by your fellow human beings.

Remember, it is your passion and compassion, the selfless sharing of the knowledge that you have received and will be receiving for the rest of your life that defines who you are. It is the giving, and acceptance, of the ultimate responsibility that has become your obligation. It is this very obligation that comes with the magnificent gift of being a healer.

This is your time—your time to take control and be proactive about your future and the rest of your life.

Or do you prefer to sit back, wait, and let stuff "maybe" happen? That is a pretty big maybe. All of the hard work, effort, energy, and time that you have put in—for a maybe? Is that what you want? Is that your future? Is it all in the hands of destiny?

Do you want your life to be shaped and controlled by people and events over which you have no say or control? Do you always want to have to react to the chaotic events in your life and put out fire after fire? Do you really want to subscribe to the limited philosophy that life is a series of never-ending chaotic events that require you to navigate through them as best as you can, and then on to the next event? Or...

Do you want to take charge, be in charge, and stay in charge of the events in your own life?

If you, like most successful people, want to be in control of your world, then you need to take charge. You need to be the one who determines what happens and what is going to happen in your life. Sorry, the technology to change the past hasn't arrived yet. So don't waste any time dwelling on the past except to appreciate and glorify the positive events that have transpired.

The way to take control of your life is to *conceive, write, direct, and star in your own movie.*

As we discussed before, it is imperative that you take a proactive attitude. You are going to make things happen *for* you; you are not going to wait for things to happen *to* you.

It really helps—no, it is a must—for you to visualize your future as you really want it to occur. If you are the quarterback, you must visualize the football sailing over the defenders and into the intended receiver's hands—before the ball is thrown. The golfer must visualize the trajectory and speed of the putt rolling into the hole before the swing is initiated. The NBA star sees the ball swishing through the net for a three-pointer long before the ball ever leaves his hands.

Conceive, write, direct, and star in your own movie.

How do you do it?

The first step is to conceive of an idea. Any idea.

In this case you might be considering or working toward a specific goal in life. To come up with an idea, especially a new idea, is the hardest part. For most people it is difficult to think beyond the reality of their daily existence.

But you are not just anyone. You have very specific goals in life.

Just by letting your mind open up and allowing it to be receptive to your subconscious, it will happen. A kernel of a thought will germinate. A mere scintillation of an idea will fester. You won't be able to grab it or hold onto it at first. But just allowing it to happen and being aware of its existence will keep it intact. It might not even be a complete thought, but you feel it and know that it is there. This is what I like to call the "seed." For after all, this initial whimsical illumination is but a seed—a seed for your future thoughts. Let it just come to you. Ruminate over it. Play around with it. Think about it as motivation and use it as the energy that will fuel your engine to move forward toward your goal(s).

As the seed germinates, it will slowly extend its roots into your conscious mind. As you play with it some more and put it into a workable context, it will form new branches, and this conscious thought will solidify.

Now comes the fun part. Visualize your thought as a reality. Visualize your thought as an *absolute* reality. Remember, great athletes visualize the completion before the action. See yourself right there, being the successful, compassionate doctor you are meant to be. Visualize where you are going now, tomorrow, next month, and in thirty years.

By visualizing your life the way you want it to be, you are well on your way to making it a reality. As Theodore Herzl said, "If you will it, it is no dream." In fact, it is these very words that initiated the foundation and creation of the state of Israel.

Theodor Herzl, Nelson Mandela, and Mustafa Ataturk had dreams. They each had a dream to establish nations that would welcome the disenfranchised. They each had a dream to create something that no one else dared to create. It was their seeds, their dreams, their visualizations that were germinated and then created.

Your thought should now be crystal clear. The seed has grown and secured itself with deepening roots. The terminal branches are now growing fruit. Just like a carefully tended tree, it is now that your creative mind will begin to bear the fruit of your vision.

Direct the greatest screenplay possible for yourself. Don't set limits. Let your mind run. Nothing is ridiculous. The Wright brothers achieved flight when everyone else thought it was impossible. Columbus set sail across the western sea when everyone else believed the world was flat and that he and his crew would certainly perish. The United States put men on the moon. "If you will it, it is no dream." These are powerful words.

Be the director of your script. Work it all out in your mind. Work with the words. Let them roll forward, tumble sideways, and even fall back a little.

Set your short-term, medium-term, and long-term goals. Write them down. Visualize them. Replay them. Visualize them some more. Conceive your future life exactly the way you want it to be. Don't be afraid. Consider all of the possibilities.

As the director, you will also want to consider other characters and circumstances. Lay out the overall foundation of your goals. Make a blueprint, chart, spreadsheet, outline, or vision board. You are the director of your movie. You can't build a house without a blueprint, and you can't effectively direct a movie without a script. This is your script.

You have to constantly monitor and adjust as you move forward. Look at your progress from different angles and viewpoints—different camera angles, close-ups, and panoramas. Be flexible with your actions and feelings as well as those of all of the other actors in your movie: premed advisors, professors, preceptors, volunteers, colleagues, interviewers, and so on.

Now go out and star in your movie. You are the protagonist. Believe in your movie, put in the appropriate effort, and you will succeed.

Your seed, your dream, has now come to fruition (now you know the root of this word). You will find new seeds within the sweet fruit. Let them germinate, and...

Conceive, write, direct, and star in new movies.

About the Author

Gary Rose, MD, FACS, is an Associate Professor of microbiology and clinical biomedical science at the Charles E. Schmidt College of Medicine in Boca Raton, Florida. He is a graduate of The George Washington University and The George Washington University School of Medicine.

Board certified in otolaryngology and plastic surgery, Rose is the author of numerous medical and surgical articles and textbook chapters. As the former Chair of the Admissions Committee of the regional campus of the University of Miami School of Medicine at Florida Atlantic University in Boca Raton and a longtime member of the Admissions Committee of the College of Medicine at Florida Atlantic University, Rose has evaluated and interviewed hundreds of medical school applicants.

A lifelong runner and certified PADI scuba instructor, Rose can be found running or diving along the South Florida coast most early mornings and weekends.

CPSIA information can be obtained
at www.ICGtesting.com
Printed in the USA
LVHW080212250719
625290LV00007B/33/P

9 781502 755919